• PRAISE FOR •

Real Moms Love to Eat

Withdrawn/ABCL

"Start with health and food—add pleasure and real life. Now you have the recipe for creating a food legacy that not only nourishes you and your family, but also uplifts the entire planet. This book gives you the blueprint for eating seductively, pleasurably, healthfully, and practically—while also feeding your family every day. What's not to love?"

—Christiane Northrup, MD, ob-gyn physician and author of the *New York Times* bestsellers *Women's Bodies, Women's Wisdom*, and *The Wisdom of Menopause*

"Beth Aldrich has written a very good primer to help you begin to make your diet an ally, not an enemy in today's time-compressed world."

—Dr. Barry Sears, author of the Zone Diet books

"Hot moms everywhere will love this book. It's easy to follow, has great recipes, and will make you laugh out loud!"

—Jessica Denay, founder of Hot Moms Club, author of the Hot Moms Handbook series

"Beth's book ignites a love affair with healthy living, offering savvy insight and wisdom. *Real Moms Love to Eat* nourishes and inspires a balanced relationship with food, from practical tips about farmers' markets to beautiful meals shared with family."

—Robyn O'Brien, author of *The UnHealthy Truth* and founder, AllergyKids.com

"This book is perfect for the busy mom who wants to stay in shape, feel good, and still enjoy good food!"

—Tracey Mallett, author of *Super Fit Mama* and *Sexy in 6*

continued...

"The ultimate mother's helper! For all of us moms seeking an answer for ourselves *and* our families, Beth reveals the secret way to get more room on your plate."

—Teri Knapp, television producer

"*Real Moms Love to Eat* is packed with tips, ideas, and recipes for today's busy moms who want fun and flavor mixed into their healthy lifestyle. Beth's energetic, no-nonsense approach makes this a perfect book for anyone looking to improve or maintain a healthy family diet—without sacrificing flavor, fun, or sanity."

—Megan Calhoun, founder & CEO, SocialMoms.com

"*Real Moms Love to Eat* gives women the opportunity to approach nutrition and wellness in a practical and enjoyable way. Beth's love for helping others become healthier and happier fills each page!"

—Joshua Rosenthal, founder, Institute for Integrative Nutrition

Real Moms Love to Eat

How to Conduct a Love Affair
with Food, Lose Weight,
and Feel Fabulous

BETH ALDRICH

with EVE ADAMSON

 NEW AMERICAN LIBRARY

NEW AMERICAN LIBRARY
Published by New American Library, a division of
Penguin Group (USA) Inc., 375 Hudson Street,
New York, New York 10014, USA
Penguin Group (Canada), 90 Eglinton Avenue East, Suite 700, Toronto,
Ontario M4P 2Y3, Canada (a division of Pearson Penguin Canada Inc.)
Penguin Books Ltd., 80 Strand, London WC2R 0RL, England
Penguin Ireland, 25 St. Stephen's Green, Dublin 2,
Ireland (a division of Penguin Books Ltd.)
Penguin Group (Australia), 250 Camberwell Road, Camberwell, Victoria 3124,
Australia (a division of Pearson Australia Group Pty. Ltd.)
Penguin Books India Pvt. Ltd., 11 Community Centre, Panchsheel Park,
New Delhi - 110 017, India
Penguin Group (NZ), 67 Apollo Drive, Rosedale, Auckland 0632,
New Zealand (a division of Pearson New Zealand Ltd.)
Penguin Books (South Africa) (Pty.) Ltd., 24 Sturdee Avenue,
Rosebank, Johannesburg 2196, South Africa

Penguin Books Ltd., Registered Offices:
80 Strand, London WC2R 0RL, England

First published by New American Library,
a division of Penguin Group (USA) Inc.

First Printing, January 2012
10 9 8 7 6 5 4 3 2 1

REGISTERED TRADEMARK—MARCA REGISTRADA

LIBRARY OF CONGRESS CATALOGING-IN-PUBLICATION DATA:
Aldrich, Beth.
Real moms love to eat: how to conduct a love affair, lose weight, and feel fabulous/Beth Aldrich
with Eve Adamson.
p. cm.
Includes bibliographical references.
ISBN 978-0-451-23558-9 (pbk.)
1. Women—Nutrition. I. Adamson, Eve. II. Title.
RA778.A43686 2012
613.2082—dc23 2011032113

Set in Sabon
Designed by Pauline Neuwirth

Printed in the United States of America

PUBLISHER'S NOTE
The recipes contained in this book are to be followed exactly as written. The publisher is not responsible for your specific health or allergy needs that may require medical supervision. The publisher is
not responsible for any adverse reactions to the recipes contained in this book.
    While the author has made every effort to provide accurate telephone numbers and Internet
addresses at the time of publication, neither the publisher nor the author assumes any responsibility
for errors, or for changes that occur after publication. Further, publisher does not have any control
over and does not assume any responsibility for author or third-party Web sites or their content.

·Contents·

V

I dedicate this book to the eight people who make me tick, who give me light, laughter and a great reason to get up in the morning. My husband and three sons have filled me up with love and purpose. My parents, brother and sister have always believed that whatever I set my mind to, I will achieve. Thank you. I love you all! I also dedicate this book to the memory of my brother, Mark, who always loved to share a good meal!

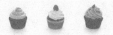

· Acknowledgments ·

L IKE A REALLY tasty meat loaf, many ingredients make up the inspiration and support of a book. My four men love me so much. They humor me when I share my ideas. They listen to my stories, eat my crazy concoctions from the kitchen, and laugh at my jokes. My husband and three sons, Tyler, Ryan, and Logan, make my life complete. Like the whipped cream on my ice cream, nothing would taste as delicious without them.

My parents, Dave and Karen, have always shared their love of food with me, from popcorn at the movies to "grandma pancakes." They joined me in my love affair with flavor from the beginning, and I love them for this and many other reasons. My brother, Mark, and sister, Michele, think I am unstoppable. My world is so much nicer with them in it.

The recipe for this book started with a conversation with my dear friend Wini. For many years she has been inspiring me to grow into the person I have proudly become; through her support and guidance, my mind has become clearer and my heart more open. My soul sister and collaborator, Eve Adamson, has a keen awareness of who I am and can channel my thoughts even before I speak them—she's a rock star mom. I love you, Eve! My nutritionist, Sherry Belcher, is my all-things-health-and-food guru. I've learned so much from her and love her candor. My quintessential friends Bonita and Caren are like sisters to me. They "get me," guide me, advise me, and love me, as I do them. My Web site editor and loyal friend, Daisy, has been more than just a friend and colleague. She has been my extra arm, my extended thoughts, and my safety net for so long. I would never get it all done without you. My assistant, Myra, is like the "front porch light on." She's always bright, shiny, and happily ready for action. She makes me look good. My good friend Falise has always supported me, helping me develop ideas and work on so many important tasks. She's a pure joy to be around. Jane Bernstein, our research assistant with the can-do attitude, made such an impact on the outcome of this book. Thanks for your flexibility, Jane.

The snowball for this book started when my dear friend Jessica Denay, who started the hotmomsclub.com Web site and has been a constant supporter of everything I do, suggested that I send my book proposal to her agent. Thank you, Jess! My agent, Claire Gerus, is one of those women you meet and instantly know that you are going to love. She's like the lucky penny in my purse; I smile when I think of her and how sincerely dedicated she is to her authors. My former radio cohost, Tracey Mallett, and former television colleague, Teri Knapp, are dear friends who know me inside and out. We connect instantly, regardless of the miles apart and their ever-present positive attitudes helped reinforce the reason why I wanted to write this book. Megan Calhoun, founder of Social-Moms.com, is virtually the best friend a girl could ever have—she's been an amazing supporter of everything I do! My friend and organizer, Molly Boren, has made space in my life for many wonderful things—lucky me. My special aunts Elaine and Mary, who have shared the countless journeys with me on this road, have always stood by my side and have always believed that with hard work, timing and patience, good things will come to me.

I am so lucky to have my dear friends in my life: Susie, Gwen, Donna, Susan, Kristie, Mary, Beth, Wendy, Petey, Michele, Ximena, Sara, and my cloned self, Kelsey, my stand-in at home when work takes me far away—I trust her and love her like a sister. To my spiritual teacher, John Douglas, thank you for your blessings and pure light and love you bring into the world. You are like the cherry on top of the aforementioned ice-cream sundae. Tracy Bernstein and the entire staff at New American Library, thank you for your patience with my countless e-mails, calls, more e-mails and more calls. I appreciate your guidance, understanding and support for this real mom who loves to eat. I hope this is the first of many delicious books we work on together!

If I didn't mention you, please know that I appreciate every person from whom I learn, and with whom I've shared and collaborated along the way. Nothing is taken for granted and I send you my deepest thanks and gratitude. *Bon appétit!*

· Foreword ·

WHAT SHOULD I eat?

This food dilemma is just one of many dilemmas facing the average mom today. Not only is she concerned about what she is eating (or not eating) but also about what to feed the family. Keeping track of our mental lists of what we should and shouldn't eat and what we would really like to eat if only it were allowed takes up a lot of time. There is so much changing advice and so many options that food choices have become a virtual landmine. How has such a simple question become so complicated? What has happened to the pleasure of eating? Does eating have to be so thought intensive?

The pursuit of health can and should be a bit more fun—and that's where this book comes in. It has practical information you can put to use right away. No matter where you are in your health goals, the step-by-step guidelines in *Real Moms Love to Eat* take some of the "boring" out of eating and bring in more fun and whimsy. And it's all about incorporating better options, not removing your favorite foods.

It's refreshing to read a book that's more about what to add to your diet than what to subtract. And, quite frankly, haven't we all had our fill of diet books? Who has the time or the inclination for a complete diet overhaul? (Besides, "going on a diet" just leads to "going off a diet" anyway!) The simple changes in *Real Moms Love to Eat* bring back the pleasure of food and the fun of eating by adding good things to your life, not the drudgery of a DIET.

As a Clinical Nutritionist for more than twenty years, I have seen how difficult it is for a woman to balance her diet along with taking care of the kids and her family's myriad needs. I commend Beth Aldrich for her fresh, fun approach to healthy eating and living. The small but significant changes over time she suggests can lead to feeling and looking better without feeling so deprived. As long as I have known her, she has had a passion for seeking out good health advice and spreading the word. The wonderful, useful information and recipes in her book can be savored one bite at a time or enjoyed all at once; just take that first step into your journey to feeling good and have fun doing it.

Healthy Blessings,
Sherry Belcher, MS, CN
Clinical Nutritionist

Introduction

LOVE TO EAT. I'm not afraid to admit it. My friends love to eat too, and you know what? I say good for us! I'm tired of hearing about all the complicated ways I can deny myself one of life's great pleasures. Food is beautiful, sensuous, absolutely delicious, and as long as we have to eat it three times or more every day, why do we make it into such a problem? Can't we just relax and *enjoy it*?

Of course, the problem is that we also want to look beautiful, sensuous, and delicious. We want to be healthy and have energy. We want to be strong and fit. As moms, we *need* to be those things, not just to set a good example for our children but to be able to get through the day and do all the million and seven things moms need to do. Our bodies and our brains need to be right on top of things, making them happen and keeping the family moving forward. That takes a lot of energy, and if you are fueling up with sugar and white flour, fake foods and caffeine, you will not be at your best.

So where is the happy medium?

It's right here, my friend, in this book. I am a busy mom but I also have learned, through my training as a certified health counselor, research, and experience, how to eat in a way that keeps me strong, healthy, energized, and slender. I'm no supermodel who lives on celery and club soda. I'm just like you—a regular mom with a great husband and super kids. And we all like to eat. Fortunately, I've discovered some pretty amazing secrets that will help you look fabulous—and *still* be able to enjoy the foods you adore.

Give me ten weeks and I'll give you a whole new food attitude . . . and a dress size you thought you couldn't wear anymore. Skinny jeans? Short skirts? Sleeveless blouses? Check, check, and check. You'll be telling the salesclerk, "Could you bring me a smaller size?"

Sound too good to be true? Think about it. Human bodies are designed to *eat*, not starve. Food runs the machine. Bodies are also designed to feel happiness and enjoy pleasurable experiences. It all goes together, a synergy created by nature. If you are ignoring it or denying it with food hang-ups and obsessions, you will end up stressed and tired and, yes, fat. It's easy to get sucked into the prevailing attitude that denial is somehow virtuous and you shouldn't *love to eat*. Forget that. You should love to eat, and your body will show you why as it starts dropping all that unnecessary baggage.

This book is both your reality check *and* your invitation to rediscover a more natural, nourishing, positive, *pleasurable* relationship with food.

The best part is that you won't be chained to a life of deprivation in order to get there. You won't be ordering the garden salad with fat-free dressing for dinner, no, ma'am, unless that's what you really want. (And is it? Is it *really* what you want?) With the Real Moms Love to Eat plan, you're going to supercharge your body and your life. You're going to embrace the pleasure, even the decadence, of really great food—and you're going to *lose weight* while you do it.

In fact, the Real Moms Love to Eat plan is so full of pleasure and fun that you might even feel like you're having an illicit affair—but this one's guilt-free, girlfriends. It's an affair with fantastic, blissful, hedonistic food, and it's going to do great things for you. When you eat smart, you'll discover that this isn't just a fling. It's the affair of a lifetime.

INTRODUCTIONS

My name is Beth Aldrich, and I am a real mom who *loves to eat*. Like you, I've always been busy taking care of my family, but I also always wondered, in the back of my mind: What is my passion? What is my life about? What am I going to *be* when I "grow up"?

The answer came, as many answers often do, in the wake of misfortune. While in a taxi, I was in a serious car accident that damaged my face. My lips as well as my hopes were smashed. I had been involved in producing and hosting a PBS TV series and publishing a magazine, and my face was one of my important assets. How could I go on TV looking like I did? That was when I began to think about what really mattered to me in life. What did I care about? What did I love? I knew I loved my husband and my kids, but what else? I was so used to just getting through the day, checking off my vast to-do list, that I hadn't spent time in years thinking about the big picture. What did I see for me? Money? Success? Fame? Power? No, suddenly all that seemed meaningless.

I began to think about the smaller things in life—the little pleasures, the momentary joys, that build on one another to create happiness. What did it all mean without that happiness, and what could I do to make that happiness easier to grasp?

Suddenly, I realized that it was a two-part equation: health and pleasure. Not just my health, but the health of my husband and my children, my friends, all the moms in the world . . . the planet itself! Not just my pleasure, but my family's pleasure, teaching my kids that life should be fun and good and happy, enjoying my friends and food and a beautiful day and all the beauty the world has to offer. Health and pleasure. What else really matters? Isn't life a waste without those two things?

I couldn't stop thinking about my hospital bed epiphany, and when I got home, I just happened to see an advertisement for the Institute for Integrative Nutrition in New York City. I had an inkling, call it female intuition, that this was the place for me. I could learn all about health, food, and, I hoped, happiness. I liked the idea of *integrative* nutrition—to me, that implied that nutrition could transform life itself. They say that when the student is ready, the teacher appears. I signed up immediately . . . and my new life began.

Once a month, I packed my bags and shuffled off to the Big Apple to study holistic health counseling and train with the likes of head teacher Dr. Mehmet Oz, Dr. Andrew Weil, Dr. Barry Sears, Dr. Walter Willett, Dr. Marion Nestle, Dr. David Katz, Geneen Roth, Deepak Chopra, Joshua Rosenthal, and many other brilliant people committed to natural health, whole food, and the pursuit of a fulfilling life. The more I learned, the more I began to see changes in myself. I got stronger, more energetic, more radiant, calmer, more aware of the influence of everything I did, more sensitive to the effects of food, exercise, and stress on my body . . . and I lost the extra pounds I'd been carrying around after my accident.

The best part of my journey was that I was able to enjoy all these amazing changes in myself *without giving up food*. I've always been a food lover. Bacon, chocolate, filet mignon, pancakes, pie . . . whatever it was, if it tasted good, I was all about it. I've always been petite, but my weight has fluctuated over the years. Suddenly, I found myself slender and strong and *still eating what I wanted to eat*! That's when I realized I was really onto something.

So that's my story, but *Real Moms Love to Eat* is about *your* story. Real moms need to take good care of themselves if they want to take good care of their families, without sacrificing the joys of life. I wrote this book for one reason and one reason only: to encourage moms like you to focus on *their* health and happiness, both equally important. Only then can you cultivate health and happiness in your children and everyone else you love.

So join me as you discover the key components of the Real Moms Love to Eat plan: step by step, delicious bite by delicious bite, you're about to get slimmer, sexier, stronger, more energetic, and better at everything you need to do each day. It all starts with the food on your plate . . . and ends with a better life.

PART ONE

Flirting with Food:

Introducing the *Real Moms Love to Eat* Plan

WEEK ONE:

The Seduction

THIS WEEK, DO FIVE THINGS:

1. Start each day with a green smoothie.
2. Eat one ounce of dark chocolate every day. It's an assignment!
3. Drink four glasses of fresh, pure water every day.
4. For dinner every night, make sure your meal contains two naturally green things, one naturally red thing, and one naturally yellow thing. (No, a bag of Skittles doesn't count.)
5. Each day, eat one portion of something you really, really desire, no matter what it is.

H, FOOD—HOW WE love you, and how we fear you. How we desire you, and how we push you away. Food, you shameless flirt, you player, you tease. You could almost seduce us into an illicit affair. . . .

And why not? Go ahead. Throw caution to the wind. This is a book about *getting involved* with food, and what better way to begin than with a good old-fashioned seduction? I know I'm not the only one who is sick and tired of being told to feel guilty about pleasure. Why should we?

Moms like us spend most of our days doing things for other people. We wake up the kids. We get them ready for school. We make sure they eat something. We send them on their way, or drive them to and from and all over town for their activities. We work outside the home or inside the home, and even after a long day of work, we still do the laundry, clean the house, help our kids with their homework, pick up after everyone, get dinner on the table (or at least bring it home and put the take-out containers on the table), and try to be supportive, encouraging, and affectionate to our husbands. We help out at school, volunteer, listen to our friends, walk our dogs, pet our cats, and—just as we've finally cleaned up the kitchen—feed everybody all over again. If we're really lucky, we get a few minutes to exercise or have coffee with a friend or watch our favorite television show.

And they tell us we shouldn't be able to enjoy a good meal? That we should skip the chocolate, cut out the fat, say no to bread and butter, step away from the bacon, and bake with artificial sweetener?

Well, I say no! I say I've had it! Are you with me? Food is pleasure as well as nourishment. It's fun, it's delicious, and it gives us what we need to move through the day, so why eat fake food or bad food or food that doesn't give us pleasure?

Yes, yes, I hear you. You want to lose weight. You want to be slender and sexy and look good in, well . . . if not a bikini (I know what a couple of pregnancies can do), at least a cute tankini or sundress.

Well, girlfriends and fellow moms, have I got a surprise for you: You can have your red velvet cupcake and eat it too. Real moms *love to eat*, and I say we deserve to eat. With a little know-how, we can eat to our heart's content and still look fabulous in the wrap dress, the high heels, or the skinny jeans. That's what the Real Moms Love to Eat plan (let's call it the RMLTE plan for short) is all about—it's ten easy weeks of fun little pleasure-invoking changes in your life that will not only help you to reembrace food the way you used to love it as a kid, but will also help you slim down, power up, and look and feel like the fabulous woman that you are.

Are you ready to make over your body and your food attitude? It's time for week one. During this first week of the RMLTE plan,

I've got five assignments for you to do each day. They aren't hard. They don't require any memorization, and there will not be a test. This is just the beginning of a long-term change in your life that will kick-start you from stressed to sensational, frazzled to fabulous, and sluggish to slenderized.

You've already seen the five things in the box at the head of this chapter, and I'll explain how to do each one shortly, so stay tuned. But first, let's begin at the beginning of every great affair: with the *seduction*.

THE PLEASURE PRINCIPLE

I don't just love eating food. I love looking at it, smelling it, thinking about it, and remembering our most passionate moments together. It's an obsession in the best possible way. Why start out talking about all the things you *shouldn't do*? Life is already full of *shouldn't*s. Tell me about the *should*s.

For instance, you *should* love what you eat. Otherwise, why bother? You *should* eat what you love. You love it for a reason. You *should* get pleasure out of a good meal, not guilt. You *should* appreciate the taste of really good, fresh, natural, high-quality food. Your body craves it, deep down, even if you've temporarily masked your natural instincts with too much fake food and junk food.

You *should* experience food with all five senses.

One of my favorite places to go is the farmers' market, because the food is so beautiful. Even if I buy just one tomato or a bunch of fresh greens, I can't help marveling at the way the gorgeous vegetables and fruits are piled on the tables or in rustic wooden crates. Real, fresh, whole food has such brilliant, sun-drenched color— bright green peppers, orange carrots, rosy tomatoes, crimson grapes, shiny red cabbages, emerald-colored lettuces, raspberries the color of a sunset, blueberries the color of twilight. . . . And you *should* appreciate how food looks when you prepare it, too—the silky shine of melted chocolate, the bronzed skin of a roasted chicken, the rainbow of a mixed green salad, the magenta-on-white of a fresh radish, the deep blush of a fresh peach or a dusky plum, the snow-white satin of cream swirled in rich dark coffee. . . . I could wax poetic forever, but you get the picture.

How food looks is just one part of the experience. At the farmers' market or even at the grocery store, touch, stroke, poke, squeeze, *feel* the food to find out what's freshest and most inviting. Pick it up and smell it too. Whether you are smelling the ripe end of a melon or squeezing the juice from an orange or reveling in the smell of bacon or baking bread or a pan of chocolate brownies right out of the oven, you *should* appreciate the irresistible aromas of real food.

Chocolate Seduction

WHENEVER I GET within a mile of the Blommer Chocolate Company factory in Chicago, you can find me with my nose to the wind, all sensors up for the smell of chocolate. Sometimes I resist because I don't really need it. Sometimes I go straight home and have some chocolate, or bake a smart version of something chocolate, like low-fat whole-grain brownies. And sometimes I'll walk right into the store and buy myself a little something. You can bet I'll take my sweet time to savor every bite.

Food has a sound, too: the sizzle of a burger on the grill, the crisp snap of a raw string bean, the juicy crunch of an apple, the exhilarating pop of popcorn. And of course, there is *taste*, wonderful taste. *You should love the pleasure of fantastic, sensual, mouth-filling, mind-blowing taste.*

Maybe because moms are so concerned with setting a good example or guiding their kids down the right path, we sometimes make ourselves feel guilty. We deny ourselves pleasure. But when it comes to food, this is a big *Oh, no, you don't!* Denial leads to obsession—the nasty kind where you can't get that bad boy out of your head and then you binge. Instead, when you give yourself the license to love a variety of foods, experiment with an array of flavors, and lighten up on your self-righteous have-to-eat-100-percent-healthy-and-be-perfect-all-the-time side, then you can give yourself permission to love—food and anything or anyone else. You find a new balance. You find your own personal way of healthy eating. Fear leads only to ruin. Denial leads to deprivation. Controlled indulgence, on the other hand, leads to freedom.

Think about your favorite food. Think about the first time you saw it, smelled it, tasted it. Think of it like a best friend—visualize the intimate details you love, the way you think fondly of a friend's dimples or silly giggle. Is your favorite food smooth, silky, chunky, tangy, salty, sweet? How do you feel when you eat it? What does it do to your body; how does it make you feel? Even if the food is something you've always thought was "bad," forget about that right now. You're in love. Think about the memories that surround the food—sometimes what we love most about food is the memory, the people, the place we associate with it.

For instance, I usually get through the day without craving sweets, but once in a while, for no apparent reason, it hits me: I must have a cupcake. Now, I just love cupcakes. They are adorable. They have power over me. They can control my car; I kid you not— like a magnet, I'm pulled right to the cupcake shop (Chicago, where I live, has plenty of choices). Or I'll bamboozle my kids into facilitating my passion: "Hey, boys, I don't suppose you're in the mood for . . . a cupcake?" Of course, now that they know about it, I can't *let them down*, so off we go.

Once I'm in the cupcake store, I'm transported: the pastel colors, the sugary smell. We all make our choice: salted caramel, black and white, cookies and cream . . . And isn't it nice how they gift wrap them for us in those pretty boxes that we tear open like wild bears? With chocolate crumbs and traces of frosting on our cheeks, we skip out of the shop together, smiling because we've shared a special splurge: *We just ate cupcakes for dinner!*

It's not like we're going to do it every day. That wouldn't be healthy or balanced. But every once in a while? Why the heck not? This is the stuff family memories are made of. As in:

My all-grown-up-but-still-loves-to-visit-his-mother son: "Hey, Mom, remember when we had cupcakes for dinner and you told us not to tell Dad?"

My husband: "You did what?"

Me: "Um . . . is that the time? My goodness, son, don't you have to be getting home to the wife and kids?"

Now, I'm the first to champion the decadent treat, but there are pleasures to be had from more modest foods too. For as long as I can remember, my dad kept a glass bowl of celery soaking in the refrigerator. When I was six years old, I would swing open the refrigerator door while chanting my oft-repeated refrain: "I'm hungry; what can I eat?" I often bumped the glass bowl while rummaging around, and I can remember the feel of those droplets of ice water splashing onto my hand and leaving a little puddle on the refrigerator shelf. I would pluck a crisp celery stalk from the bowl, swing the door shut, and begin chewing before I'd even stepped out of the kitchen. I loved it—the snap, the crunch, the watery saltiness, even those juicy strings, plain or dipped in creamy ranch dressing. I still love celery. I add it to salad; I have it for a snack; sometimes I even eat it for breakfast. I like to get a lot of bang for my bite, so I look for bites that will fill multiple senses at once. Cupcakes, celery—in my mind, it's all good.

Another thing I'm into these days is roasted salmon. I love the rich flavor, buttery, tender texture, and the knowledge that it is giving me the important omega-3 fatty acids my body needs. I wouldn't care quite so much, however, if it weren't so beautiful and delicious and if it didn't have such a positive effect on how I feel after I eat it, supplying me with sustained energy and emotional fulfillment for hours afterward.

Some of my passions are so brazen that I almost feel embarrassed. I love ice cream and I'll eat fruits and vegetables all week long, anticipating an ice-cream indulgence on the weekend, but recently, smack in the middle of the week, I got a hankering. Before I knew what I was doing, I was walking straight into Cold Stone Creamery and ordering a small cup of cake-batter ice cream with Heath bars, bananas, almonds, and caramel.

What was I thinking? It was Tuesday, for goodness' sake! Guarding my little cup as if it were made of gold, I slunk to the back of the shop and savored each magnificent candy-, nut-, and fruit-studded bite. Oh, the ecstasy . . . the afternoon delight! The door opened and another customer walked in and I swear I blushed, turning my face aside. Could any one woman deserve such pleasure? What would the neighbors say? But oh, what a lovely fling it was. . . .

Foods I'm Loving Right Now

WE ALL GO through food phases. Right now I've got quite a list of my current favorite foods. I'll show you mine if you show me yours!

- Grilled onions
- Charleston Chew candy bars
- Grilled cheddar sandwiches
- Kettle-cooked potato chips with French onion dip
- Any kind of hot-fudge sundae with whipped cream and salty nuts
- Steamed lobster and warm drawn butter
- Crisp apples with creamy peanut butter
- Chocolate cream pie with chocolate shavings (I scoop off the shavings and eat them last)
- A big, fat, juicy hamburger with mayonnaise, ketchup, yellow mustard, onion, and pickles
- My special-recipe kale salad with cumin and olive oil (for the recipe, see page 209)
- Green protein smoothie with a side of Ezekiel raisin-bread toast and butter
- Fresh stir-fried chicken with pea pods, carrots, broccoli, and onions
- Pepperoni-and-onion pizza (nobody else in my family likes onions—wanna share with me?)
- Kashi Autumn Wheat and Cinnamon Harvest cereal with vanilla rice milk
- Blue Moon beer with an orange slice
- Tortilla chips and fresh salsa with extra onions (I'm seeing an onion theme emerging here—my breath smells fine; I swear!)
- Turtle candy (my dad and I both love these)
- My best friend Bonita's no-bake brownies (So healthy, I eat them for breakfast—for the recipe, see page 75)
- Angel hair pasta with meatballs and red sauce
- Chicken Parmesan drowning in red sauce
- Ginger chicken with ginger-soy reduction sauce
- Raspberry chicken from *The Silver Palate Cookbook*
- Spring greens with goat cheese crumbles, pistachios, and fresh roasted beets

Another passion of mine right now is raw lasagna. That might sound strange to you, but it's really delicious. Thinly sliced zucchini strips stand in for noodles, and my favorite part is the cashew "cheese," made with raw cashews, sea salt, and lemon. Fresh basil and oregano, sun-dried tomatoes, and a beautiful raw tomato sauce finish off the dish. It may be good for me; it may be full of natural enzymes and antioxidants; it may be totally raw, vegan, and politically correct; but what matters most to me is the fantastic, amazing, multilayered taste. I find myself stealing swipes of cashew cheese from the food processor, scooping it up with stray zucchini slices before I even get the whole thing into the pan. Every time I make this recipe, it brings back memories of going out for pizza with my family when I was a little girl. Of course, it's not what I ate back then, but the sensual experience is the same, a memory trigger that makes the meal all the sweeter.

The point is pleasure, girls. Remember what you love. We moms get so used to denying ourselves what we most desire that remembering the pleasure inherent in our earliest food experiences, not to mention more recent ones, can make food seem like a friend, not an enemy. Even when we say we're splurging, we're doing it with guilt and telling ourselves we're doing something wrong, or we do it in front of the television and forget to notice what we're eating! What a waste. Recapturing the pleasure of food is the important first step—then we can go back and measure out our pleasure so it doesn't become gluttony, but instead adds color and spice to our lives. Out with the guilt and excess weight; in with the happy!

FOOD NOSTALGIA

In that spirit of recapturing your childhood sense of pleasure about food—back before you associated food with guilt, denial, binging, and other negative feelings—let's take a look back at *your* early food memories, when food was just plain good old happy food. Think about your earliest and most positive food memories. What did you love to eat as a kid? Don't even think about whether you *should* eat it now. No censoring your desires! It's no crime to remember—and no calories, either. Was it chili dogs at the drive-in? The taste of just one more mini candy bar on Halloween night after you had already brushed your teeth? Your mom's sweet-potato casserole with marshmallows melted on top?

When I think back, I remember lying in bed on a Sunday morning, slowly awakening to the smell of bacon. I would imagine the aroma, like a cartoon cloud circling over my bed and teasing me awake. My father was cooking, and I knew that at eight a.m. sharp, breakfast would be ready: his famous fresh orange juice whipped in the blender, his paper-thin crepes (we called them Grandma Pancakes—for the recipe, see page 260), and, of course, the much-anticipated bacon. My brother and sister and I looked forward to those breakfasts every week—and why shouldn't I still? I still enjoy bacon every now and then. I just limit how much bacon I eat.

Growing up, I had a healthy relationship with food. I ate what I wanted and was very clear about what I didn't want. Like any child, I was a picky eater: Salmon? Gross. Beets? Grandma food. Green vegetables? I don't *think* so. Now that my palate has matured, I love all those foods, but I remember standing in front of the open refrigerator door, nibbling a slice of American cheese and wondering why the adults preferred cheese that stinks. Even so, I was always willing to try something new. Food was fun and food was interesting, a collection of colors, shapes, and textures that could turn out to be anything: creamy, salty, crunchy, sweet . . . and could also link up with any emotion of the moment, becoming ally, enemy, nurturer, energizer, friend. Food was important . . . as it *should be.*

I remember buying my first cookbook as a young woman living alone for the first time, *The Silver Palate Cookbook* by Julee Rosso and Sheila Lukins. I sat in a comfortable chair and thumbed through the crisp pages, amazed at the potential—all those delightful, exotic recipes! I could almost smell and taste the food as I read the ingredients. I loved the way the book was organized, with its dainty illustrations. I still have the book, and many of the pages are earmarked, testament to how often I've used it and how many of the recipes I've prepared since that day. One of my favorites is the Mango Chutney Chicken. I remember reading that recipe for the first time and thinking, *How the heck is all that cayenne pepper going to taste mixed with mango chutney and syrup?* It was so easy to prepare, and lick-the-plate delicious.

Did you have a favorite cookbook? Food magazine? Did you like to flip through your mother's recipe box? When you think back, don't just think about what foods you loved—think about the context, the people involved, the places, the *feeling*. Food can be a powerful connection to family memories and traditions, and just the thought of it, not to mention the aroma, can stir up emotions that we then attach to the food. This can bring back powerful positive feelings—and negative ones too, if you have some food memories that aren't so great. Those are worth remembering too, but for the sake of this exercise, focus on the positive ones.

Did your family grow a garden? Did you help pick out food at the supermarket? What tastes did you love the most? Was food a reward for something you did well? If you ate the foods you didn't like, what foods did you get to have afterward? Vanilla ice cream with chocolate syrup? Your favorite cake? A second helping of macaroni and cheese?

You will probably find that many of your early food memories center around comfort foods that aren't traditionally considered healthful today, but that's just fine. I want you to find your most pleasurable food memories—soon enough, we'll get around to helping you relive slimmed-down versions of those positive memories with all of the pleasure and none of the guilt. For now, just kick back and remember.

Understanding the emotions we all have connected to food—many of which stem from childhood—can help us understand that food can have power over us. However, it also gives us power over food, because we can go on to use that food in a way that sustains and fortifies us. We can use it for sustenance, for pleasure, for energy, even for entertainment, as long as we are using food, and not the other way around. When we begin to understand food's influence in our lives, we can then become skilled at transforming dinner into something more meaningful—something that can have a direct impact on how we look and feel. A great meal can leave you feeling better than when you started, especially when you focus on the pleasure aspect and use it to your advantage. For instance, take what you love and tweak it so it enhances everything you love about yourself. That can be your high standard for every single bite you take. It can be full of pleasure *and* help make you look and feel your best. Your fond memories and food pleasures become assets to your health and well-being, rather than liabilities. It's all in how you reenvision the food experience. I'll teach you how throughout this book—in fact, I'll start right now, with the five things I'd like you to do this week. Are you ready?

DO FIVE THINGS

Are you beginning to feel seduced? Excellent. Now, don't get carried away. Let's begin with five simple assignments—these are all about pleasure and energy, so I'm sure you'll want to jump right in. I'm not going to batter you over the head with *shouldn't*s. No, these are things you *should* do, so embrace them with all the passion you would throw into any torrid affair. After all, it's *food*. And you *love to eat.*

1. START EACH DAY WITH A GREEN SMOOTHIE.

What could be easier than kicking off the morning with a sweet, smooth, thick, ice-creamy smoothie? Whether or not you are a smoothie person, I would like to make a case for the power of the smoothie. What you eat at the beginning of your day can influence your energy level all day long, and that is powerful. I've tried a lot of breakfasts in my day, from pancakes and bacon to miso soup and tofu. My professional opinion, after a lot of research as well as personal trial and error, is that no breakfast will power you up and make you feel good all day long like a green smoothie with a scoop of protein powder. It's your new magic bullet.

Now, maybe you're thinking, *Smoothie, okay, I can maybe handle a smoothie . . . but a* green *smoothie?* Green is gorgeous! Green is energy. Green is your power secret. Just because you aren't used to drinking a sweet, fruity smoothie that happens to be green doesn't mean you can't start now. The magic of the smoothie is its ability to hide nourishing ingredients that you might not normally eat . . . and it can still taste like fruit or chocolate! Yes, fruit or chocolate. Or both! The green in a smoothie comes from healthy raw greens, whether you buy them in powder form or throw a handful of freshly picked and washed greens from your garden or farmers' market into the blender.

The taste of raw greens can be potent to some, but in a smoothie, their taste mellows due to the addition of the fruit you add to them, such as a frozen banana or a handful of raspberries, or cocoa powder. It's a sort of bait-and-switch dietary trick you play on yourself—and the perfect way to introduce more greens into your diet. While it may take a seasoned green smoothie drinker to consume a "greens-only" smoothie, you'll want to keep adding more greens once you develop a sincere longing for the energy and good feelings you get from a green smoothie. Eventually, you'll even start craving the taste of those greens! Just start by combining greens with sweet fruit flavors and juice, so your body and taste buds will adjust to the distinct flavor.

When I began my green smoothie routine, I started gradually, just because greens are very detoxifying. To be blunt, I was using the restroom a bit more (my new flat belly thanked me), but my skin and eyes were clearer, and I experienced amazing bursts of energy throughout the day. At first, I just added a dash of the green powder, but as I got used to the taste of greens with my fruit, I added a little bit more each day. I worked my way up gradually to the full scoop of powder or, when they are in season, a full handful of fresh leafy greens, and sure enough, my body adjusted to the physical changes and interesting new flavors. I would watch the green smoothie spinning in the blender and smell that aroma of green until it became something familiar that I started to crave every day.

In short, greens can have a strong taste, but fruit chills out the whole experience into a sweet sensation you're going to love, and as you ease your taste buds into it, you'll be able to enjoy more and more and more greens, until you're practically bursting with gorgeous energy. Habit is a powerful thing, so don't give up. This is your chance to feel amazing every morning.

So do yourself a favor. Start each day this week with a green smoothie. If you don't like it, you don't have to do it after this week . . . but how could you not like it? You can mix any flavors that appeal to you, and you'll start to look and feel more fabulous. Here's how to do it:

🍳 GREEN SMOOTHIE

In a blender, combine:

1 frozen banana or ½ cup frozen berries (strawberries, blueberries, blackberries, raspberries, etc.) **Note:** Use frozen fruit to make the smoothie fluffier and smoother, like a milk shake—you'll get the consistency of ice cream without all the fat and calories.

1 cup fresh organic juice (apple, orange, pineapple, etc.), nonfat milk, soy milk, almond milk, coconut water, or water

1 scoop powdered raw greens (find them in the health food store) or one handful fresh greens, like baby lettuce, kale, Swiss chard, spinach, or beet greens (or work up to this amount)

1 scoop protein powder: whey, rice, hemp, or soy protein are good choices that you can buy plain or flavored

1 tablespoon ground flaxseeds

A few ice cubes, if you want your smoothie to be even thicker and more ice-creamy

OPTIONAL FLAVORING: 1 tablespoon peanut or other nut butter, 1 tablespoon raw cacao or cocoa powder, 1 teaspoon instant coffee, ½ teaspoon vanilla or other flavored extract, dash of cinnamon

OPTIONAL SWEETENER: 1 tablespoon agave nectar, real maple syrup, brown rice syrup, or granulated raw sugar

Experiment with different flavor combinations until you find ones you love. Orange juice with strawberries? Bananas and peanut butter? Cocoa, cinnamon, and coffee? Raspberries and vanilla? No matter what the flavor, you'll know you are doing your body a big favor—and your body will return the favor with positive energy. You'll practically have a halo.

2. EAT ONE OUNCE OF DARK CHOCOLATE EVERY DAY. IT'S AN ASSIGNMENT!

It's simple. It's delicious. It makes you feel pampered and decadent and a little bit naughty. And it's *crucial for survival*! Okay, I made up that last one, but still, chocolate can make your day, and if you are like me, the lack of it can break your day. That's why the second thing you have to do during week one of the RMLTE plan is to eat one delicious ounce of high-quality dark chocolate *every day*.

No, don't try to get out of it. You're not weaseling your way out of this one, my friend. This one is serious. This is *chocolate*.

Part of the myth surrounding chocolate is that if it tastes so good, it must be bad for your health, but that's totally untrue. When chocolate is mixed with tons of fillers and cheap processed sugar, well, then it's not so great for you, but high-quality dark chocolate *is*. Cacao, the source of chocolate, contains antibacterial agents that fight tooth decay. Seriously! Your dentist can *get behind chocolate*. (Of course, the sugar in chocolate does mean you still have to brush your teeth afterward.)

Not convinced? Fine, here's more:

* The smell of chocolate may increase theta brain waves, resulting in relaxation. I can testify to this one.
* Chocolate also contains phenylethylamine, a mild mood elevator.
* The cocoa butter in chocolate contains oleic acid, a mono-unsaturated fat that may raise good cholesterol.
* Drinking a cup of hot chocolate before meals may actually diminish appetite.
* Women who eat chocolate live a year longer, on average, than those who don't.
* The flavonoids in chocolate may help keep blood vessels elastic.
* Chocolate has been known to increases antioxidant levels in the blood.

* Mexican healers use chocolate to treat bronchitis and insect bites.
* The carbohydrates in chocolate raise serotonin levels in the brain, resulting in a sense of well-being in most people.
* The best news of all: Recent studies all over the news say that a small amount of dark chocolate every day may actually reduce your risk of heart attack and stroke.

Isn't chocolate great? Isn't it amazing? I agree! I buy a high-quality bar of dark chocolate at the health-food store and have one square each day. Choose your time. Midmorning? Midafternoon? After dinner? It doesn't matter when you do it. Just one square. Just do it.

3. DRINK FOUR GLASSES OF FRESH, PURE WATER EVERY DAY.

Chocolate may not actually be required for survival, but *water is*. Water keeps all our systems running, and it is also a key to clear thinking, great skin, and de-bloating.

I learned the importance of water for physical functioning early on. I vividly remember one freezing winter day when I was training for a marathon with a twenty-mile run. Every time we ran past our cars we'd stop and get a drink from the water bottles we'd wrapped in blankets to keep them from freezing. I can still taste the room-temperature water going down my throat as I guzzled from my water bottle. I could feel how essential it was. Nothing can beat the satisfaction.

When you start drinking more water, you will also need to use the bathroom more often, but your body will soon adjust. So drink up, girls!

4. FOR DINNER EVERY NIGHT, MAKE SURE YOUR MEAL CONTAINS TWO NATURALLY GREEN THINGS, ONE NATURALLY RED (OR BLUE OR PURPLE) THING, AND ONE NATURALLY YELLOW (OR ORANGE) THING. (NO, A BAG OF SKITTLES DOESN'T COUNT.)

My favorite way to accomplish this item is *always* to add a salad to lunch and dinner. Chop up tomatoes, red and yellow peppers, red onions, green beans, peas, cucumbers, zucchini, summer squash, green onions, maybe even a tablespoon of corn, or whatever you have in the crisper or find in the store or farmers' market that is fresh, seasonal, and looks irresistible to you. I like to top my salad with some brightly colored fruit too, just to make it pop with surprise flavors. Try strawberries, blueberries, sliced plums, or orange sections. Drizzle with your favorite dressing and voilà—your to-do is done.

5. EACH DAY, EAT ONE PORTION OF SOMETHING YOU REALLY, REALLY DESIRE, NO MATTER WHAT IT IS.

What do you really, really love? Whatever it is, quit feeling guilty and enjoy it *today*. Just one portion—that's all you need to get the pleasure without going crazy. For instance, I am a bread junkie. Top it with butter and I am your slave for life. I know how carb- and fat-filled buttered bread is, but when I really want it, I'm going to have it. But I'm not going to eat the whole loaf—the trick is to have it in a smart way. I treat bread with butter like dessert. If we are going out to eat somewhere that has amazing bread, I will have a light supper—some lean protein and greens or vegetables—just so I can save room for some bread. But if I feel more like dessert that day, I'll skip the bread. (However, if you should ever find yourself in Rome—or Paris—or a dinner party at the home of a fabulous cook, don't hesitate . . . go for both. Just eat light at the next meal.)

Love your food and hold it to your highest standards. Experience it and know how to work it in your favor. Have a little bit, and enjoy the hell out of it. Every woman I know has some kind of entangled love affair with food, but I say, *Brava!* Your affair shouldn't be a one-night stand or a gluttonous binge, however. Instead, it can become a lovely, long-term, balanced, nurturing-because-it's-rational sort of relationship. What you eat and how much of it you eat can make you better or it can make you worse, so remember that before you take a single bite. It's not about indulgence versus denial. It's about pleasure and vitality and *life*— one portion at a time.

I like to think of eating well, for pleasure and radiant health, like having an affair with your own husband. You know he's good for you, so you bring back the joy, the excitement, the *flavor* of your first exciting encounters. You can trust him. Food isn't a quick fix, a fling—it's a marriage, but it can stay spicy forever. Savor each delicious bite and crave more.

WEEK TWO:

Make It All About You

THIS WEEK, DO FIVE THINGS:

1. Get back in touch with your individual desires, preferences, and passions by making a list of your ten absolute favorite foods.
2. Get to know yourself even better by taking a good hard look at the ten foods you really do dislike the most. (Guess what: *You never have to eat them again!*)
3. Explore your adventurous side. Make a list of five foods you haven't tried but would be willing to try.
4. Drink five glasses of fresh, pure water every day.
5. Drink up! Upgrade your favorite beverage today.

OU DON'T HAVE to tell me: It's all about the kids. It's all about the husband. It's all about work. The pets. The house. The volunteering. Guiltily, you might squeeze in an hour at the gym or yoga class once a week, or the occasional pedicure while catching up with your girlfriends while making the grocery list while answering e-mails on your iPhone while texting your kids about when you have to pick everybody up today.

And no matter how much you keep your chin up, it probably seems that most of the time, it's not about *you*.

It's so easy for moms to put everybody's needs, desires, and preferences first. You make what your husband or your kids like to eat. You go to the places they want to go. You do things to facilitate their lives. You want to make them happy. But what about you? Girlfriend, you deserve—no, you *require*—a little more self-regard.

So this chapter is about you—gorgeous, fabulous, savvy, powerful you. I know you still have to do all those other things, but if you don't carve out some space for yourself, it will begin to chip away at your own health and sanity, and then you won't be any good to anybody. So do it for them, if that's what it takes, but this week, I want you to really focus on you: what you love to eat, what you love to do, and even what you can't stand and shouldn't ever have to tolerate.

CHANNELING YOUR INNER CHILD

Think back to when you were a little girl. I mean it. Think back right now. Stop reading, put the book down, close your eyes, and remember a happy time from your childhood, or not even a specific time, but just how you felt in your own body. Think about running, jumping rope, playing hopscotch, lying under a tree or on the beach, or sitting in the sun. Remember how you felt before you started worrying about everybody else. Think back to when you were twelve, or eight, or five. How far back do you remember?

Think about what you used to do when you were lying on your bed, looking at the ceiling, imagining all the things you might do someday. Remember swinging on a swing, playing tag or keep-away or kick-the-can with your friends, the feel of the air at twilight in the summer, the rush of jumping off the diving board or coasting on your bike down that big hill—look, no hands!—or just running as fast as you possibly could. Think about how you saw the world and what you hoped for and dreamed about. Think about how *light* you were, how little you cared about what all the grownups were doing (*so* boring!), how much you loved to move and laugh and spin and jump off things, climb a jungle gym or do cart-wheels or somersaults or just roll down a grassy hill.

Close your eyes and think about it. Not the tough times, not the scary times, but the good, free, joyful times. Think about how you felt in your body, the spark in your soul. Feel it inside—it's still there, even if you haven't thought about it or accessed it for years. Go ahead. Let yourself drift a bit. I'll wait.

Are you there? Do you feel it? Can you remember? If not, that's okay. Some people find this exercise really difficult. If it helps to pull out old pictures of yourself as a child, try that. Look at yourself and try to connect with that younger you. If you still aren't feeling it, no pressure. No worries. Just keep thinking about it, and see if you can get there this week—even if you just get a glimpse, a tickle, a momen-tary thrill that takes you back. Even if you can remember only one perfect moment, find it and bring it back up to the surface.

This is a VIP exercise—in other words, it has a Very Important Point. The reason I want you to get back in touch with the way you felt as a child is that the child you were still lives in you, and de-serves just as much love and affection, empathy, and consideration as your own children. You deserve it now, *from yourself.* When you can feel that inside you, that nurturing, motherly feeling toward yourself, you will be better able to understand how important you are, how much you should let yourself feel pleasure—and how much you should avoid hurting yourself by not giving your body what it needs. Would you ever consider feeding your children or talking to your children the way you sometimes feed and talk to yourself?

In some little way, we can all be our own mothers. We can even spoil ourselves a little. Just to see our own smile in the mirror, or just a little unfurrowing of that take-it-all-on brow. Because that's *you* in there, and finding your way back to yourself, beyond your to-do lists, responsibilities, and *should*s, will help you get back to what you really love about life, about yourself, and about food.

FOOD FORAYS DOWN MEMORY LANE

Speaking of food . . . let's get even more specific. I'd like you to go back into your memory now, and think about your earliest positive experiences with food. What did you love to eat as a child? Don't judge yourself. If you loved canned ravioli or hot dogs or cotton candy at the park, then that's what you loved. What were your absolute favorites, the things you would save your allowance to buy after school, the things you would beg your mom or dad to let you eat? Cinnamon toast? Cherry tomatoes out of the garden? Popcorn with butter at the movie theater? Bubble gum at the swimming pool? That special cheesy potato or green-bean casserole your grandma made on Thanksgiving?

When I think back, I remember Sunday-night dinners at my grandmother's house. I can still feel exactly how I felt back then, anticipating that weekly trip. My brother, sister, and I would pile into the car with our parents and drive to Grandmother and Grandfather's house. We knew what we would get to eat, and we couldn't wait: Grandmother's mouthwatering roast beef, roasted or mashed potatoes, and tender string beans. The meal wasn't always exactly the same, but it always *felt* the same because it was surrounded by ritual. We'd pull up into the driveway, scramble out of the car, kiss and hug our aunts and uncles—we were the only grandchildren for a while; cousins came later—and then we'd go inside and head straight to the crystal candy dish Grandmother always had filled with colorful ribbon hard candy, Red Hots, or some kind of seasonally appropriate sweet. My sister, brother, and I would each sneak a single piece before dinner, when nobody was looking. I'm confident all the grown-ups must have known exactly what we were up to, but nobody ever said a word, because it was Grandmother's house and Grandmother's candy dish, and in her home, the grandchildren were on a slightly longer leash.

Grandmother had her rules, and none of us children dared cross her, out of pure respect that she commanded with her natural style, grace, authority, and, of course, her special skill in the kitchen. I remember the day she decided to teach me how to set a table properly. I watched her every move like a hawk. I marveled over the shiny silver utensils, her manicured nails precisely positioning the knives, forks, and spoons. The aroma of slow-cooking beef permeated the air. I can still smell it, and feel the silver in my hands as I practiced placing it correctly.

It was my grandfather's job to put on the oven mitts and place the roast beef on the counter. Grandmother said the meat had to "sit" to let the juices "sink in." She would cover the roasting pan with a tent of aluminum foil, something I still do today. We would all wait expectantly, hovering near the kitchen but not daring to get in the way. My grandfather would sharpen his carving knife, then slice the tender meat, the pink juices streaming down the sides. When the slices of meat lay on the serving platter like a perfectly toppled line of dominoes, garnished with a sprig of rosemary, Grandfather would bring the platter to the table. On the other side of the kitchen, Grandmother would add the butter to the whipping bowl of potatoes and dribble in the milk as she whipped them with the mixer. Next came the green beans and the freshly baked dinner rolls. Then, and only then, did we sit down, give thanks, put our napkins on our laps, and pause for a moment to admire the perfectly aligned silverware, the sparkling wine goblets filled with chilled water and dripping with dewy condensation, and the gorgeous, savory spread of our dinner.

I remember exactly how every dish tasted. The first bite of roast beef was always so rewarding, so reliably the same. I still don't know whether the food was so good because it was simply that good, or because it was all part of the ritual, the family togetherness, the safe comfort of my grandparents' home. It doesn't matter. What matters is that it was my favorite meal of the week, and one of my favorite memories to this day.

Think back to your favorite meals. Think beyond the food to where you were, who you were with, and the rituals or traditions that surrounded the meal, whether it was just Popsicles on the front porch with your best grade-school friend, or something as fancy as an elaborate holiday meal with your entire extended family.

Another reason I want you to think about your favorite meals from childhood is because I want you to recognize when the environment surrounding a meal made it so much better. When you share food with people you love in a lovely place, every bite is special. You don't need to overeat or emotionally eat or stuff in food you don't really like when everything about the meal is thought-out and beautiful. Every time you eat, you can make it an event, a ritual, and an act of love. Every meal can be memorable, and when you treat food with that kind of respect, you treat yourself with respect, too. And you'll be making memories for your own children.

WHAT'S YOUR PLEASURE?

Now that you're back in touch with your inner child, let's think about who you are now, and what you love now. What gives you the greatest pleasure? Maybe you aren't even sure. How long has it been since you ate something you really wanted, not because it's good for you or you know it has this or that vitamin or mineral or antioxidant, not because it's on your diet plan, and not because it's *not* on your diet plan and you know it's forbidden and you are feeling rebellious? When was the last time you ate something you really wanted, only because you genuinely, deeply preferred it?

When you spend most of your time focusing on what other people need, it's easy to forget what you actually want, but getting back in touch with your genuine preferences and desires is essential to conducting a successful love affair with food.

So let's think now about what really gives you pleasure. What do you love to eat? Some of the things you love may be linked to childhood. When I was a child and I had a friend sleep over, my mom would always make Rice Krispies Treats, and that would always make us so happy. It was such a special ritual that marked the sleepover as "official." Later, when I was pregnant with my third child, I had a total obsession with Rice Krispies Treats. For weeks I made a pan every single day—an entire box of Rice Krispies, an entire bag of marshmallows, all the requisite butter. I would melt it all together and press it into the pan and then promptly eat them, or cut them into squares and hide them, hoarding them from everyone. My husband tried to take one of those treats once. He says it was like at the amusement park when the ride attendant tells you to keep your hands and feet inside the car at all times during the ride, only in his case, it was, "Keep your hands and feet away from the pregnant lady and her Rice Krispies Treats at all times, or she may bite them off!" I even brought them to the hospital with me when I went into labor. In fact, that morning I took the time to bake a pan of brownies, so all my extended family members visiting me and celebrating the birth of my third son would have something to eat—and would therefore keep their hands off my Rice Krispies Treats! The thing I love most about this memory is that my third son is crazy about Rice Krispies Treats, and whenever we get the chance, the two of us share them.

Sometimes, however, the things we love come to us later, and that's just as valid a passion as the food preferences that are rooted in childhood. Growing up, I wouldn't have anything to do with beets. Disgusting! I remember my grandmother scooping them out of a glass jar or aluminum can onto a plate with a *swish-plop*. To me, the very sight was horrifying. I just couldn't handle that bloodred color. Gross. But I grew up and one day a friend offered me a roasted yellow beet from her salad plate at lunch. Hesitantly, I tried it . . . and everything changed. Now I *love* beets! I enjoy that sweet, earthy taste in salads, roasted and topped with a pinch of sea salt and a drizzle of olive oil, sometimes tossed with chunks of fresh oranges, or scattered over mixed greens with goat cheese, walnuts, and balsamic vinaigrette. Yum! Nutritious, full of vitamin C? Sure, but that's not why I love them. Now I can gaze at that deep, intriguing ruby color with genuine fondness. It's as beautiful as a lush glass of rich cabernet. If eating beets is for grandmas, then just call me Granny.

I'll have you making some lists this week, but for now, just start thinking about what foods really give you pleasure, and which foods you only think you like because you are supposed to like them—or supposed to avoid them! For some people, the quickest way to a craving is to tell themselves they can't have something. If you decide you can't have sugar, then what's the first thing you have to have? Probably the first sweet piece of junk food that happens to capture your attention, even if you don't really love it. That stale birthday cake in the office refrigerator that didn't even interest you yesterday is suddenly irresistible as soon as you aren't supposed to eat sweets.

So be honest. Be frank. And be happy. When you know what you really love, you are opening the door to the very best kind of healthy eating.

BUILDING A BETTER BODY

This book is, obviously, about food. (Your first clue was probably my obsessive enthusiasm about the stuff!) However, making it all about you is also about your body and your health. I would feel remiss if I didn't take a few minutes to remind you that eating is a way to take care of yourself, but it's not the only way.

You depend on your body for everything. When it doesn't work, nothing works. That's why you absolutely, positively must take care of yourself. Remember your inner child? Nurture that little girl! Your body is constantly changing (think puberty, pregnancy, perimenopause, and menopause), and at each stage, it needs different things, both nutritionally and in terms of exercise and self-care. I think a lot of women aren't necessarily in tune with what their bodies need or what's going on. But if you think about it, you can feel what seems to work and what doesn't.

For example, let's consider exercise. We all know (or so we've heard) that exercise is good for us. It keeps our muscles strong, it's important for a healthy heart, and it supposedly boosts our mood. Maybe it does that for you, and you won't get through the day without your daily run. But if you are grumpy instead of pleased when you get home from the gym, something is wrong; maybe you worked yourself *too* hard, or maybe you are sleep-deprived and should have taken a nap instead, or maybe you didn't eat well enough to support that workout, or maybe you are busy and stressed and you really didn't have time for it that day. I can't tell you how often I am driving down the road in Chicago and I see a woman huffing and puffing, running and sweating and looking like she's about to faint. If you love running, you go, girl; but if you hate it, then you aren't listening to your body. You aren't taking care of yourself. If you hate what you are doing, then I can guarantee there's a better way to get your cardiovascular fitness.

You don't have to work so hard to look and feel good; I promise you. When your body is in rhythm with the inner you, then your body will become what it is supposed to be: in balance.

Instead of worrying so much about burning off every ounce of fat that jiggles, I'd like you to think about your hormones. Seriously.

What goes on inside your body is an amazing, practically magical, impossibly complex chemical extravaganza, and when it works, it works whether you do that two-hour kickboxing class or not. But if one of those many hormones gets off-kilter, then watch out. You'll start feeling bad. Hormones have a huge influence on how you feel.

HORMONAL HARMONY

The primary hormones that affect moms are cortisol (the so-called "stress hormone"), estrogen, progesterone, and (believe it or not) testosterone. The interplay of these four hormones can make you feel energized, strong, and healthy, or depressed, anxious, panicked, and angry. It amazes me how much hormones can influence a woman's entire perception of herself. That's why you have to get your hormones balanced before you can really feel well enough to do anything else about your health. When your hormones are in check, your energy flows freely and you will naturally be able to maintain a healthy weight (with the help of the Real Moms Love to Eat plan, of course).

When you experience stress, your body releases cortisol. An elevated cortisol level can increase your appetite and, more specifically, can make you crave sweets and simple carbs like chips and cookies. Give in to those cravings and you'll cause a spike in your blood sugar and then a drop, which will make you crave even more sugar and simple carbs. All those extra calories result in extra body fat, usually stored deep inside you, around your internal organs, pulling on them and making it harder for them to function. They clog up your blood and slow everything down. A woman filled with cortisol and fat is like a car filled with dirty oil.

It's a vicious cycle, and a lot of diets will tell you that you have to just stop eating the sugar and carbs, but the problem with that is simple: If you don't first stop the release of the cortisol, you won't be able to stop those cravings. They are like a freight train. What are you going to do, stand on the tracks and wave your little arms? I don't think so. Are you going to tell that miserable child inside you that she can't have a cupcake, or are you going to try to help her feel less miserable? I vote for option number two.

You have to stop the release of the cortisol first—by giving yourself a break, slowing down a bit, or at least practicing some serious stress management intervention, like *gentle* exercise, yoga, stretching, deep breathing, or more time for yourself. (Can you up those seasonal pedicures to monthly pedicures? When was the last time you had a massage? Are your girlfriends wondering whether you dropped off the planet because you haven't seen them in so long?)

Fighting cravings when cortisol is already working its evil will on your brain is just too hard. I'll talk about reducing stress periodically throughout this book, but let me just say here that *reducing stress is absolutely essential for reaching your ideal weight.* When you calm down, the cravings calm down, and then you can make better decisions about what you really want to eat. Nothing you know about food will help you until you get your stress under control.

The other thing I would like you to do, especially if you have been experiencing unexplained increased symptoms of stress, like insomnia, irritability, weight gain, cravings, bloating, depression, anxiety, joint pain, and irregular periods, is to go to your doctor and get a full hormone panel, including a full thyroid panel (TSH, T3, and T4). At some point, your hormones will begin to fluctuate in preparation for menopause, and even if that's a decade or more away, a full blood panel will give you a baseline by which to measure hormonal changes as they occur. The more you know about your hormone levels, the better armed you will be to work with your doctor to keep them in balance. I highly recommend that you keep a file of all your hormonal and blood workup results, so you can refer to them later.

Balanced hormones make for a balanced mom.

I did this recently. I consulted with Dr. Pamela Smith and had a complete blood panel and saliva testing done. When she saw the results, she prescribed a compound thyroid medication and a compound progesterone, and wow! I began to notice changes within a couple of weeks. To determine the correct prescription for my body, I retook the evaluative tests a couple of times over the course of a few months. Through the process of elimination (and with a lot of patience), we were finally able to balance my hormones, and when that happened, everything started happening! I was carrying around some extra weight, and it just fell off. I had been so tired, and I perked right up. It's not that the hormones fixed everything— it's that when the hormones were fixed, *I* was better able to make the right choices for my body and myself.

DO FIVE THINGS

How are you feeling now? Real moms know not to just answer, "Fine," like a robot. Think about it. Are you feeling a little more empathy for yourself? A little more commitment to doing what's best for you? A little more interest in what's going on internally? Great. Now it's time for your weekly assignments. You've already been thinking about these things, but now I want you to write them down. So get out your Real Mom notebook (you *do* have a Real Mom notebook, don't you? No? I'll wait while you find one, buy one, or make one. Mine has flowers on the cover) and get ready to make some lists. These are lists that are *all about you*, so do your best and be honest. You're going to need this information later.

1. GET BACK IN TOUCH WITH YOUR INDIVIDUAL DESIRES, PREFERENCES, AND PASSIONS BY MAKING A LIST OF YOUR TEN ABSOLUTE FAVORITE FOODS.

In the past, whenever I would go on a diet, I would get so frustrated because of the foods that I couldn't eat. I'd silently sit and read the diet to myself, shaking my head once I got to the part of the book where the author explained that some of my favorite foods were *not* allowed on the plan. *Okay,* I thought to myself, *but in two weeks, I can eat my favorite foods again, so I guess I can follow this diet, lose some weight in time for summer/that wedding/my class reunion/ bathing suit season, and then go back to reality.* Well, the smarter, more logical side of me now knows that this is madness. It's unrealistic and it wreaks havoc on your metabolism (we'll discuss the very important metabolism piece in a later chapter). I want to live my life not by a strict plan, but on my terms. I want to eat what I want to eat, enjoy it, *and* look fabulous for summer/that wedding/my class reunion/bathing suit season. I want that to *be* reality.

But before you start writing down your ten favorite desserts, let's think about what it really means to have an absolute favorite food.

While I was studying at the Institute for Integrative Nutrition, the recurring theme shared by all of our guest instructors was, "Listen to your body." The key proponent to working with a holistic nutrition counselor (and following the guidance in this book) is to find what works for your own mind and body. We all have bioindividuality, and that means that foods that agree with me and that I prefer will probably be different from foods that agree with you and that you prefer. The current trend is to turn to a prescribed diet plan for a list of what to eat or not to eat, but only you and your body know what your list should contain. The answer is inside you.

For example, if I were to list my top ten favorite foods right now, I might be tempted to just start listing desserts. However, if I think about it and how I feel before, during, and after I consume them, my list might change. Some nights, I'll lie in bed regretting a meal choice I made for dinner, as I hold my stomach trying to wish away the indigestion and gas pains. But that never happens after a clean raw salad or bowl of fruit. So what is my body telling me? It's telling me that I have to really *think* before I list my all-time favorite foods. It's about what I love to eat not only for how it tastes, *but also* for how it makes me feel.

To put it in more passionate terms, you can give in to a whim and have a torrid one-night stand with a rich, decadent dessert, or you can flirt with it a little and then go back to your wholesome lifestyle. Flirting is fun, but eating well feels great. So as you make your list, remember that you can have the best of both worlds.

Keeping that in mind, here is my list of all-time favorite foods . . . as of this moment. (My list might be different tomorrow—because it's a mom's prerogative to change her mind!)

1. Beth's Kitchen Sink Salad (baby and romaine greens, goat cheese, tomatoes, scallions, carrots, chopped almonds, broccoli, green, yellow, and red peppers, apple slices, and a homemade balsamic vinaigrette dressing)

2. Lobster with drawn butter
3. Protein-rich pasta and marinara with meatballs (I love Dr. Barry Sears's protein pasta and Dreamfields' low-glycemic pasta)
4. Sexy Raw Lasagna (see recipe on page 92)
5. Raw Nut Pâté (add recipe cross page 91 served on lettuce with tomato and green pepper)
6. Chocolate of any kind (Little-girl Beth doesn't care what kind, but wise grown-up Beth knows dark is best)
7. No-guilt hot-fudge sundae (made with Luna & Larry's Coconut Bliss frozen dairy and soy-free ice "cream," organic hot fudge, Truwhip nondairy whipped topping, chopped almonds, and a real pitted sweet cherry)
8. Grilled steak burger with sautéed onions served between Bibb or romaine lettuce leaves, no bun
9. Grapefruit from my mom's hybrid grapefruit tree (sweeter than anything I've ever eaten). No sugar necessary!
10. Ginger Chicken (chicken tenders sautéed in a reduction of olive oil, soy sauce, powdered ginger, and rosemary) and sautéed Brussels sprouts with onions

Wow, I'm getting hungry. Now it's your turn! Take a quiet moment and think very carefully about what you really love—you *and* your body. And don't feel married to your answers. You can always change them tomorrow. Your cravings are yours alone, and you will begin to see patterns of eating habits and desires, even if today you adore raspberries and tomorrow you much prefer ratatouille.

Write down your ten favorite foods and save the list, not just for inspiration when you want something to eat but you aren't sure what. You'll also want to refer back to this list later, as your tastes change and evolve. You might be surprised, a few weeks from now, how much your list will change. As a health counselor, I can tell you that when people start acknowledging what they really like and really want, exclusive of what anyone tells them they should like and want, they develop a clearer, saner, more rational perspective on what to eat. They begin to pinpoint, through trial and error, which foods really work best for them, and that's part of the reason that your list might be and can be ever changing. You are con-

stantly evolving and growing and learning more about who you are
and what you love . . . and, most of all, what your body needs.

2. GET TO KNOW YOURSELF EVEN BETTER BY TAKING A GOOD HARD LOOK AT THE TEN FOODS YOU REALLY DO DISLIKE THE MOST. (GUESS WHAT? YOU NEVER HAVE TO EAT THEM AGAIN!)

I didn't want to go here right away—after all, I don't like to
dwell on the negative. However, I think it's time. I think you're
ready to go over to the dark side. The scary place. The place where
it lives. You know what I mean. *It* is the food you can't stand, that
fills you with dread, terror, *horror* (*eek eek eek!*).

We all have those childhood memories of the things we had to
eat that we could just barely choke down. The things we secretly
fed to the dog under the table. The things we kept in our cheeks,
then spit into the wastebasket when we got up to get a "glass of
water." (As if our mothers didn't know!) Do you remember sitting
at the table long after everyone else had gone away because you just
couldn't choke down that last bite of now-clammy asparagus or
okra or watery boiled spinach?

My nemesis was my mom's "famous" sliced-hot-dog-potato-
and-onion casserole. She would sauté the hot dogs (seriously, should
the words *sauté* and *hot dogs* even appear in the same sentence?)
with sliced potatoes and onions. I can still smell that distinct odor.
Ewwwwwww. The funny thing is, I can go to a ball game at Wrig-
ley Field and enjoy a hot dog covered in onions and mustard with
the rest of the fans, no gag reflex at all, but slice 'em up and sauté
'em in a pan and you lose me—in fact, I'm running at top speed in
the opposite direction.

Even as a young girl, I thought hot dogs and bologna only
vaguely resembled food. I was always suspicious of their strangely
homogenous texture and fleshy color, and I rarely ate them. Today,
as an adult, I realize that I don't *have* to eat them. In fact, it's probably better for me if I don't.

I've found much better options, like all-natural, chemical-free
chicken sausages. I love them, and I've even managed to find a way
to enjoy them *sliced* and *sautéed* (I guess the apple doesn't fall far

from the tree). I don't add potatoes and onions, but I might add some scallions, minced fresh garlic, and chopped kale and serve them over whole-grain pasta. Still, I think my mom would be proud.

Another food that I just couldn't stomach as a child was Brussels sprouts. My mom would boil them—that's how housewives made Brussels sprouts back then—and serve them up, fully expecting us kids to devour them just because she and my grandfather shared a taste for the noxious, stinky little balls of green. But c'mon, Mom. No butter, no salt, nothing (*shiver*)? As an adult, I've discovered that (ironically) *sautéing them with onions* in a little olive oil brings out their nutty sweetness and they're practically lip-smacking. Even my kids like them.

Why on earth do adults think children would enjoy mushrooms or eggplant? Slippery, slimy, and way too earthy for a young palate, they really are grown-up foods, although I must confess (and you're probably going to think this is weird): I have never ever eaten either one. And I have no intention of ever doing so. So there!

That's the beauty of the next list: The foods you dislike are yours to dislike, and you never have to eat them. Nobody can make you. Your mom did what she could, but if she was never able to get you to like Brussels sprouts or broccoli (or hot-dog casserole), well, her nutritional authority ended when you moved out and got your own kitchen.

So here is my list of deal breakers, gross-out foods, the stuff I simply don't like and you can't make me eat. And don't tell me I can't like it if I haven't tried it. I absolutely *can* not like it and never try it if I darn well please!

1. Mushrooms
2. Eggplant
3. Traditional hot dogs (sliced and sautéed . . . with . . . *urp* . . . onions and potatoes . . .)
4. Snails (even if you call them escargot)
5. Tomato juice (I love tomatoes any other way, but get that juice away from me.)
6. Avocado (Not by choice—this food gives me severe stomach cramps.)

7. Squid, calamari, and oysters. They may be three different foods to you. To me, they are all the same: eek!
8. Black olives. I plan never to let one squeak against my teeth again, and I'm a better woman for it.
9. Coffee (Calm down. I didn't say *you* had to dislike it!)
10. Cheesecake (Once a year, I eat this on my father-in-law's birthday; he loves it, and out of love and respect I struggle through it. Next time, you can share my slice.)

Now it's your turn. As your holistic health counselor, I forbid you to dislike exactly what I dislike. Get your own list! Figure out what you really, really can't stand, write it down, and then decide (gloriously) that you will *never touch the stuff again.*

3. EXPLORE YOUR ADVENTUROUS SIDE. MAKE A LIST OF FIVE FOODS YOU HAVEN'T TRIED BUT WOULD BE WILLING TO TRY.

The world is filled with food, and chances are, you haven't tried most of it. In fact, most people eat just a few foods most of the time—their favorites, the ones they know how to cook, the old reliables they know they like. However, diversity in your diet isn't just nutritionally beneficial. It can also open up whole new worlds of pleasure and appreciation. So let's think about the foods you've never tried, or even the ones you haven't tried for years because you think you don't like them. And let's consider giving them another shot.

Even though I have "jumping out of an airplane" on my bucket list, I'm not sure when I'll actually do it. I say explore your adventurous side, but only in ways that you are willing. As I confessed in the last section, I've never tried mushrooms, but I'm not *that* adventurous. I mean, hurtling through the atmosphere strapped to some guy with a parachute is one thing, but *mushrooms?* I have to draw the line somewhere.

I remember years ago, going to dinner with my friend Kelly, when I confessed that I had never tasted salmon. Her salmon looked awesome, and I asked if I could possibly have a small bite, just to try it.

She was absolutely taken aback. "You've never tasted salmon? Oh, you're going to love it, especially the way it's prepared here." I can still taste it as I type this page . . . pan-seared, the exterior was crisp and the tender fish was slightly sweet, buttery, flaky. Much to my surprise, it didn't taste fishy at all (and never should, just for your information). In fact, it was so tender and satisfying, it's now one of my favorite foods. I hadn't realized what I'd been missing all that time.

As I mentioned, I couldn't stand the sight or smell of Brussels sprouts, but that all changed after my trip to Paris with my cousin. We wanted to go out for a special dinner, so I asked our hotel concierge for a good restaurant referral. After a forty-five-minute cab ride, we pulled into the circular drive of a gorgeous white house with bright lights shining through the windows reflecting off the neatly manicured landscaping. Once inside, we were seated at a quaint small round table topped with a cream-colored tablecloth, elegantly adorned with a simple small vase containing two white roses. Given that the menu was written in French, I had a bit of a time ordering, so I decided to ask the waiter to request that the chef create a meal for two hungry American women.

I was a little worried about what the final bill would be, since we'd given the chef free rein like that, but I decided that, hey, you only live once, and I'd always wanted to say I had eaten at a fine French restaurant in Paris, so I decided to just go with whatever happened.

Our first course arrived at the table; a beautiful salad containing fruit, greens, nuts, and a tasty cheese whetted our appetite for our main course. The sliced steak filet topped with a savory-sweet wine reduction sauce looked delicious. But what was this? Brussels sprouts? Wait a minute. I hadn't signed up for Brussels sprouts . . . or had I? I thought about requesting a different dish, but I didn't want to be the difficult American. As I moved the suspicious little sprouts around with my fork, I realized they actually looked tasty. Throwing caution to the wind entirely, I dug in, and by the end of that meal, I was discreetly licking the back of my fork and almost licking my plate. Those Brussels sprouts, roasted and smoky-sweet, were just about the best vegetable I'd ever tasted.

Chocolate mousse cake topped with whipped cream and a cup of tea wrapped up the meal, and I was supremely satisfied—not just because I could check "fine French meal in Paris" off my list, but because I had tried something new, and it was *worth the risk*!

There are still plenty of foods I haven't tried yet, but now that I have gotten more adventurous, here are five foods I might be willing to try . . . even if I never make it back to Paris:

1. Red snapper. (Is it as good as salmon? Maybe I'll find out.)
2. Rabbit meat. It's very popular in Europe. I don't know why it hasn't caught on here. If I ever get the chance, I'll give it a try.
3. Abiu, a fruit that grows in Brazil, Ecuador, Peru, and Venezuela. I hear it grows on trees more than one hundred feet tall, and has a bright yellow skin and a pulp that tastes like caramel. I love the taste of caramel. Plus it's rich with vitamins A and C. There are just so many delicious fruits around the world that most Americans have never even heard of—I want in!
4. Frog legs. After years of reading the Frog and Toad series of books to my sons, I might have a difficult time eating these, but I think I'd try it once. Because don't they taste just like chicken?
5. Cactus fries. These are cooked pieces of cactus that have been sliced and covered with a flour-cornstarch mixture before being deep-fried. I don't make a habit of eating deep-fat-fried food, but I think it would be interesting to try just one.

So what's on your list? Write down a few things you think you might be willing to try, whether they are unusual or just something you've never quite been able to brave. Even more important, start noticing the foods out there in the world that you've never tried. Look especially to ethnic cuisines. Have you ever been to an Ethiopian restaurant? What about a Vietnamese restaurant? Have you tried much German food, or any dishes from South America? What about Australia? Open your mind to the great big world of food out there, and you might just become a little more well-rounded . . . not to mention a little smaller waisted.

4. DRINK FIVE GLASSES OF FRESH, PURE WATER EVERY DAY.

I'm one of those people who just loves drinking water. I always have some with me. When I'm thirsty, I crave nothing more than fresh, pure, lightly chilled water. I know not everybody is such a fan of water, and I know plenty of women see those recommendations out there to drink eight to ten glasses of water every day and roll their eyes. When you aren't used to drinking water, that's a heck of a lot of water.

But water is so important for your health, beauty, and energy level that I'm asking you to start with a more modest goal. Drink five glasses of pure filtered water each day this week—that's one in the morning, one after breakfast, one with lunch, one with dinner, and one in the evening. And just one more glass than last week. Just one cup each time—you can do that; I know you can. Throughout the RMLTE program, you'll gradually increase the amount so your body can get used to it, although you probably will need to hit the restroom a little more often than usual this week. But that's okay. Consider it internal cleansing! Like I told you last week, your body will adjust. Plus, when you drink more water, you may notice you aren't hungry quite as often. Maybe when you thought you were hungry, you were really just thirsty.

5. DRINK UP WISELY! UPGRADE YOUR FAVORITE BEVERAGE TODAY.

I used to be a serious diet-soda drinker. I drank it every day. I also drank sugar-sweetened iced tea and sugary juices, and I'd wonder why I couldn't lose weight. I had no idea that I was drinking almost a full day's supply of calories in beverages alone—and I thought that I was being so good by drinking diet soda!

Beverages are one of the most common diet traps. Whether your weakness is regular soda or diet soda, energy drinks or just way too much fruit juice, this week I'd like you to take a serious look at what you drink and how you can upgrade.

I'm not saying give anything up that you really love. No way. This is all about you and your pleasure, and I totally understand having your favorite things and clinging to them with ferocity!

(Like me with my Rice Krispies Treats.) Instead of thinking about deprivation, I want you to think about how you can indulge yourself *even more*, by going for pleasure rather than caving in to a bad habit.

If you are a coffee drinker but you use the cheap canned stuff, think about swapping it for some really good whole-bean, organic, fair-trade coffee, or coffee in a decadent flavor, like hazelnut, vanilla, or crème brûlée. If your upgrade is more expensive, consider finding a balance by drinking a little less. A little bit of a great thing is always better than a whole lot of a mediocre thing, especially when it comes to food and drink.

If you love soda, think about how much lighter, better, more energetic, and *classier* you will feel if you swap even one of your daily sodas for club soda with a splash of fresh juice. Or lighten up your morning OJ with club soda and a wedge of fresh orange. Yum!

I love juice but I was drinking too much before. I still drink it—juice is a beautiful thing! It comes from nature and is filled with a high concentration of nutrients that your body can quickly absorb. Freshly squeezed juice is also filled with live enzymes that are easier to digest than whole fruit. Enzymes found in fresh fruits and vegetables have the important job of converting food into body tissue and energy. Enzymes also help increase metabolism, and that's a good thing! I advise you to drink fresh juice, but juice it yourself if you can, or buy it freshly juiced, and just have a little bit. The stuff in bottles and cans sitting on the grocery store shelf doesn't count. You might as well be drinking soda. But even with fresh juice, you don't need much. Fresh juice still contains pure "natural" sugar and can result in too many calories if you drink too much of it. Whole fruit is always the best choice, but when you really want juice, make it excellent and fresh, and savor every drop (we'll talk more about juicing in an upcoming chapter).

I upgraded my juice to freshly squeezed, and now I drink just a few delicious ounces in the morning, so I have a chance to use that juicy energy during the day. (Although my all-time favorite beverage is filtered, pure water with a slice of fruit or a few ripe berries swimming around in it.)

Make Your Body a Diet-Soda-Free Zone!

IN CASE YOU don't already know this, I will tell you, in my capacity as a holistic health counselor, that artificial sweeteners are *bad* for you! I repeat, they are bad for you! If this book facilitates any changes in your diet, I hope crossing diet soda off your list of daily liquids is one of them. I can't believe that I still see people guzzling diet soda, even though they know about the dangers of artificial sweeteners. I guess it really is addictive, but this is an addiction worth breaking.

There are countless studies outlining the harmful side effects of artificial sweeteners. Just to name one I read about recently, in an article published in the *Journal of Neuropathology & Experimental Neurology*, John W. Olney, MD, of the Washington University School of Medicine in St. Louis, notes that animal studies reveal high levels of brain tumors in aspartame-fed rats. According to Dr. Olney, recent findings show that aspartame has mutagenic (cancer-causing) potential, and the sharp rise in malignant brain tumors coincides with the increased use of aspartame. That's just one of a bunch of studies that show or suggest how harmful artificial sweeteners can be. I don't doubt that artificial sweeteners can cause cancer in humans, but even if you do, I always say that when it comes to safety in food ingredients, if there is any doubt, then please go without!

If you are a tea drinker, consider upgrading your tea of choice. Right now my favorite tea is green tea. Plenty of research suggests that green tea lowers cholesterol levels and might even inhibit the growth of cancer cells. To sweeten the pot, my new passion is stevia, a no-calorie sweetener derived from the leaves of the stevia plant that is available in liquid or powdered form. Stevia has very few calories, so it doesn't adversely affect blood glucose levels. Stevia has a regulating effect on the pancreas, and it actually helps stabilize blood sugar levels, lowers blood pressure, and increases energy. For me, green tea with stevia is a definite upgrade from my old go-to diet soda.

Finally, consider that some of those beverages you are swilling are probably just not worth the price. What can you give up that you don't really love, and that isn't serving your best interests? Remember, this is all about *you*. When I realized my sugary tea and soda habits were just that—habits—I ditched them. I wasn't really attached to them, so now I never drink diet soda or sugar-sweetened beverages at all, and that means hundreds of calories saved that I can spend on something more worthwhile.

Making your diet as well as your lifestyle *all about you* isn't nearly as selfish as it might sound. You are the hub of the wheel that is your family, and you can't afford to break down or limp along at minimum efficiency. You are *everything* to your kids, so you owe it to them, as well as to yourself, to operate at your peak. And that means taking care of *you*. So get with it, find your inner child, and take care of her. And that's an order!

Now that you're two weeks into the Real Moms Love to Eat plan, I'm betting you are feeling pretty great. Keep going with the plan—next week will be even more transformative, so stick with me, keep loving yourself, and get ready to tackle some of your more, shall we say, *dysfunctional* dietary "friends."

WEEK THREE:

Make Over, Salt, Fat, and Sugar, (Your Dysfunctional Friends)

THIS WEEK, DO FIVE THINGS:

1. Give processed food the boot and upgrade your table salt. The more intense flavors in gourmet salts help you use less.

2. Buy three new herbs or spices and start using them on your food. I'll introduce you to some of my favorites and tell you what they can do for you *and* the food on your plate.

3. Banish evil trans fats from your home for good. Swap out all trans fats (hydrogenated and partially hydrogenated oils) for olive oil, canola oil, and the occasional worth-it splurge of real organic butter.

4. Get rid of sweet nothings like high-fructose corn syrup and white sugar in your diet. They are *not* your friends. Trade up to better sweets. And OMG, you aren't still drinking diet soda, are you? Stay tuned for another tirade.

5. Drink six glasses of fresh, pure water every day.

OH, GIRL, IF a fellow Real Mom doesn't break it to you, who will? I've heard the rumors. You've been hanging around with the wrong crowd. I know, I know, those friends of yours are *fun*. Hanging around with them is like a party, twenty-four/seven. Indulgent. Decadent. Sure, they may be a little dark, a little edgy. You may know, in the back of your mind, that they are *bad news*. But they make you feel so good in the moment.

And then there's the hangover.

By now, perhaps you've recognized that I'm going with an extended metaphor here, but the fact is that there are some food ingredients that really are like dysfunctional friends, the ones you think have your back but really don't, the ones who comfort you only while it's convenient and then turn on you when you are at your most vulnerable. They seem innocent enough, but when you hang around with them too often, they spell trouble.

I'm talking about salt, fat, and sugar.

It's all right. I understand the whimper escaping your lips. You can cry on my shoulder. I'll cry with you. Because I *love* salt, fat, and sugar too. Who doesn't? Salty chips and movie popcorn, thickly buttered bread and crispy french fries, chocolate-chip cookies and birthday cake and that secret stash of M&M's in your purse? You don't have to tell me! Does a woman really even *know love* before she's tasted a chocolate truffle or a really great cupcake?

Alas, overindulging in salt, fat, and sugar can spell the end of smart eating and a svelte waistline. Like your craziest girlfriends who convince you that it really is a good idea to do just one more round of tequila shots or go skinny-dipping in the hotel pool (the one with the twenty-four-hour security camera), salt, fat, and sugar can get you into some serious trouble.

Now dry your eyes, because here comes the good news: Real Moms *can* eat salt, fat, and sugar. You don't have to ditch your dysfunctional friends. You just have to limit your exposure to them—or better yet, give them a makeover.

Fortunately, making over these dietary black holes can be not just easy but delicious and satisfying. Because let's face it—you're not going to totally ditch your crazy girlfriends, and you're never going to totally give up the three things that make food so irresistible. When you limit yourself, however, to the very best salt, the most heart-healthy fat, and the best whole-food sweeteners, you really can have your cake and eat it too. I have complete faith that you can manage your dysfunctional friends without letting them bring you down.

So here's the key: When you eat salt, or fat, or sugar, make it the *good kind*. Make it *worthwhile*. Make it *count*. Only then can your deepest desires be truly satisfied. Only then can you move on with your life. Here's how to dig in and make it happen.

SALTY SEDUCTIONS

What's so evil about that cute little saltshaker? Nothing, really. The real danger from salt comes from processed food, which is sometimes so packed with sodium—the ingredient in salt that causes your body to hold on to water, putting more pressure on your circulatory system—that too much can trigger a whole cascade of health problems that Real Moms absolutely do not need to deal with. You've got too much to do! You don't want to add "manage high blood pressure" to your list, do you? Wouldn't you rather take a few easy steps to prevent the problem instead?

High blood pressure, a.k.a. hypertension, is practically an epidemic in the United States, according to many health experts. Although Real Moms are all young at heart and beautiful, each in her own way, we should all be aware of the dangers of hypertension. Scientists estimate that as many as 90 percent of Americans will become hypertensive in their lifetimes, and epidemiological studies show that the prevalence of hypertension is correlated with the amount of salt in the diet. While scientists don't totally understand the full extent of the link between salt and hypertension, and the occasional study claims the link is tenuous, most research supports the connection.

Another study published by the American Heart Association recently found a link between a high-salt diet and insulin resistance, a precursor to diabetes. Yikes!

So for health, energy, and, quite frankly, for a flatter, unbloated tummy, Real Moms shouldn't be salting it up like there's no tomorrow. The American Heart Association recommends 2,300 milligrams of sodium per day for young healthy people, and less than 1,500 milligrams per day if you are middle-aged or older or already have high blood pressure. And that's not a lot of salt.

But stress and worry can elevate your blood pressure too, so instead of wasting the rest of your week wondering whether you're on the verge of a medical emergency, make an appointment with your doctor for a checkup and have your blood pressure taken. Or go to one of those blood pressure machines they have in some stores. One reading isn't necessarily accurate, so take your blood pressure a few times, and then about once a month to monitor it. A normal blood pressure is less than 120/80. (These numbers are a measure of pressure in the heart when it is beating and when it is relaxed between beats.) If your reading is normal, quit worrying. If it's higher than normal, give your doctor a call.

In the meantime, there's a supereasy way to cut almost all the salt out of your diet. It's just this: Quit with the processed food, already!

Even a simple, innocent-looking can of soup can contain a full day's supply of sodium or more. Why do that to yourself when it's so easy to make soup? (In fact, you'll find some great recipes in part three.) Cutting out processed food, or at least cutting down on it, will make such a difference in your sodium intake that you'll be able to salt your homemade food without worrying even a little bit. The American Heart Association also recommends checking the labels on any processed food and avoiding those foods with more than 200 milligrams of sodium per serving. That's an easy number to remember, right?

Personally, I prefer home-cooked food every time. It tastes great with perhaps a sprinkle of salt. A frozen microwavable "diet" meal, on the other hand, is full of way more salt than you would ever want to eat, and it *still* doesn't taste good. So Real Moms, the choice is clear: Make fresh food at home, enjoy the taste more, feel healthier and more like you ate actual food, lower your blood pressure, and banish your belly bloat. I see no downside.

The Easy Way to Fight Hypertension

WHAT'S SO GREAT about a baked potato, a sweet juicy peach, tender roasted beets, a succulent red tomato, a creamy banana, or a rich, buttery avocado? These fresh fruits and vegetables contain a lot of potassium, which combats hypertension, balances sodium, and fills you up with food that is decidedly *not* processed. Load up on the plant foods and you will help your body thrive in so many ways. You might not even miss the salt.

Now, back to that little ol' saltshaker sitting there so innocently and cutely on your dining room table, all gussied up to match the pepper grinder. What exactly do you have in there? If it's regular table salt from the grocery store, then it's time to consider an upgrade.

Ever since I can remember, I've loved the flavor of salt, and I salt everything. I'm one of those annoying people who salts her food before even tasting it. (I'm *really trying* to break that habit!) But because I'm such a salt lover, I also consider myself something of a salt connoisseur. I can definitely taste the difference between ordinary processed table salt and gourmet salt, such as Himalayan salt or sea salt.

But the problem with table salt isn't just the inferior taste. Salt is a mineral that comes from the earth or the sea. The way nature makes it, it has a nutritional benefit. However, regular old white table salt, like white flour, is highly processed and totally stripped of the beneficial minerals and trace elements that it originally contained. It's also likely to contain aluminum as a drying agent, and I'm not eager to ingest any more of *that* toxic metal than absolutely necessary.

Sea salt, on the other hand, is typically produced through evaporation, leaving more of the trace minerals in the salt, such as iron, calcium, and potassium. It's unrefined in the very best sense. I think it tastes much better than table salt, with a more pleasing flavor. You can usually find it in a coarse or fine grind. In my opinion, the best kinds come from France and aren't completely white, due to the trace minerals. The kind harvested by hand is the least processed. Yum!

Other salts are better for your body too. Here are some to try:

* **KOSHER SALT:** This salt is purer, cleaner, and freer of additives than regular table salt. It has less of an unpleasant bite and it's also less salty than table salt, containing less sodium by volume because of the shape of the granules.
* **HIMALAYAN PINK SALT:** One of my favorite salts, this salt has a rich, savory flavor and pretty pinkish hue, thanks to lots of potassium, iron, magnesium, calcium, and copper. It comes from (obviously) the Himalayas, and it is what lives in my cute little saltshaker at all times.
* **FLEUR DE SEL:** This delicate, flaky salt rises to the top of the salt ponds in the Guerande region of France. Harvested just once a year, fleur de sel is considered the cream of the salt crop. Use it on top of fresh greens, vegetables, and meat. Don't waste it in cooked dishes. It's a delicate, lacy, very special sprinkle for your most cherished dishes.
* **GRAY SALT:** Sometimes called Celtic sea salt or *sel gris*, gray salt comes from France and contains healthy magnesium.
* **BLACK SALT:** Sometimes called kala namak, this unrefined mineral salt from India or Pakistan has a taste of sulfur and can do a magic act on scrambled tofu, making it taste like eggs. It's also a classic ingredient in Indian cuisine and even in Indian medicine, where it is sometimes used as a digestive aid. It isn't actually black. I would describe it as more pink or mauve.
* **RED SALT:** Sometimes called Hawaiian sea salt, this reddish salt has an earthy flavor.
* **SMOKED SALT:** Oh, delish! Smoked salt is literally smoked in cold smokers over wood fires, so it adds a lovely smoky flavor to foods, no grill required. A real treat when you can find it.
* **WHATEVER YOU FIND!** There are many different gourmet salts out there. Just look for natural, unrefined salts rich with minerals, and your taste buds may never tolerate plain old table salt again.

Finally, reducing salt is much easier if you find flavor in other places—namely, with herbs and spices. When you cook with onions, garlic, pepper (black, white, red), spices like cumin and cinnamon, and fresh or dried herbs like rosemary, basil, and oregano, everything tastes more exciting. You need only a tiny sprinkle of salt to bring out the best in highly flavored food.

I love to use herbs and spices, but I didn't always know how to do it. Much comes with practice. Start slow, adding just one herb or spice to a simple food like grilled chicken or fish or rice. As you get to know each taste, you'll discover what you like and dislike. Then you can get more daring, combining flavors.

Here are some of my favorite herbs and spices:

* **GARLIC:** It just makes everything taste better (with the possible exception of desserts!). Fresh, minced, crushed, ground into a paste, powdered, crystallized, whatever. You don't need to use a ton and give yourself garlic breath. A sprinkle will add flavor without overwhelming.

* **GINGER:** Pungent and refreshing, ginger is a staple in Asian foods, and ginger tea or just chewing on a raw slice is a great way to calm a queasy stomach.

* **CUMIN:** My current fave spice. I love the flavor it gives my Energy Kale Salad (recipe on page 209).

* **CAYENNE PEPPER:** A natural for spicy foods, cayenne can surprise you in other realms too. Try just a dash to liven up lemonade, or to add spice to brownies or hot chocolate. Cayenne pepper is good for your circulation.

* **CINNAMON:** It has a compound that can help stabilize your blood sugar. It's great in baked goods, of course, and in some savory dishes, like Cincinnati chili and Indian food. I love a dash of cinnamon in my smoothies.

* **ROSEMARY:** I have a rosemary plant in my garden that grows like a weed, so I sprinkle the feisty little spiky leaves into all my savory dishes. I like to toss a sprig into the pot when roasting meat, or I'll sprinkle the leaves on Ginger Chicken (recipe on page 222).

* **BASIL:** When celebrity chef Rick Bayless was a guest on my PBS TV series, *For Her Information,* he suggested I buy fresh-cut basil in the grocery store, place the stems in a glass of water, and when they sprout roots, plant them in a

small window box or planter. What a great idea! Basil is easy to grow, and you can pull off a leaf whenever you need that intoxicating flavor.

Herbs and spices are so interesting that you'll discover whole new worlds of flavor. You may even forget all about that little old saltshaker. At least until your next batch of popcorn.

IN-FAT-UATED

Simple, indisputable fact: Fat has more calories per ounce than protein or carbohydrates. If you eat too much fat, you can end up eating too many calories, and that's how you gain weight. However, before you plunge into fat-free fanaticism, consider the upside of fat. Fat keeps you feeling satisfied longer. You can nibble on fat-free cookies all day and rack up thousands of calories you wouldn't have eaten if you had had just one regular cookie made with real butter. In fact, even if fat has more calories than carbohydrates, you may be more likely to *get fat* by eating too much sugar and starch. That's right: Fat-free can make you fatter than fat-full.

The problem with fat is that it tastes so good that Real Moms who have trouble saying the n-word (that's *no*, as in, "No, thanks, I don't want another helping of macaroni with double cheese," or, "No cookies for me, thanks; I'm saving my appetite for dinner") can end up eating too much fat. It's just so irresistible.

It's not that we feel compelled to eat sticks of butter. It's what fat *does* to food that makes us fall in love. Adding fat to sugar or starch makes both of those substances harder to resist. For example, every time I go to the movies, that intoxicating aroma of movie popcorn almost makes me swoon. I forget what movie I'm going to see. All I can think about is a big bucket of popcorn I can share with my sons. I always surreptitiously stick out my tongue to capture a few salty-buttery-crunchy bites before I even hit the seat. When somebody protests, "Mom, don't start eating it until we sit down!" I pretend I don't hear a thing. It's popcorn-induced selective hearing impairment. That's my story and I'm sticking to it.

Would I love air-popped kernels, naked of salt and fat? No way. I'm a Real Mom, not some pretend-perfect mom who measures out half-cup portions of the plain stuff to stick in my purse before the movie. What's next, carrot sticks and radishes during the Sunday matinee? I don't think so.

But it turns out that the mysterious yellow liquid the cineplex likes to call "butter" is some pretty nasty stuff. And extreme. Real Moms need to know their good fats from their bad fats. For example, one report I read said that a large "buttered" movie theater popcorn can contain up to *four days' worth* of saturated fat. Gulp.

But here's what will really kick you in the arteries: Saturated fat is bad, but trans fat is even worse, and depending where you get your movie popcorn, that bucket could be loaded with this worst-of-the-bad-fats junk. Trans fats don't occur in nature, and our bodies don't really know what to do with them, so they build up and build up until our organs get all clogged up. Considering heart disease is a major health hazard for women, this is a serious consideration. Trans fats can wreak havoc on your health.

Unless you've been living in a cave, you've probably heard that trans fats are bad. Maybe you've heard that most (food-savvy) countries in Europe have banned them. But what are they?

Trans fats are those fats labeled as hydrogenated or partially hydrogenated. They start out innocently enough, as vegetable oil, but then they are treated with a chemical process whereby they are heated and subjected to hydrogen bubbles. The vegetable oil takes on some of the hydrogen, changing its consistency to make it more solid, like lard. It looks more like butter that way. It tastes more like butter that way. But butter it ain't.

In the final stages of trans fat creation, the hydrogenated oil is steam-distilled to remove the foul odor. That makes it shelf-stable. It won't start stinking the way rancid butter or oil would, but make no mistake: It's old and disgusting and evil.

Trans fats do a real number on your health. Some people like to say that eating a steady diet of trans fats is just as bad as smoking, and just as likely to be the (literal) death of you. We know they interfere with your metabolic function, and we know they can raise your cholesterol to extremes previously unknown by mere saturated-fat eaters. In other words, trans fats are *bad, bad, bad*. Some nutritionists claim they could instigate heart disease, cause cancer, or just make you really, unnaturally fat. The last thing Real Moms want to do is fill their families up on the stuff. So what's a movie-popcorn-lovin' Real Mom to do?

Fortunately, lawmakers have begun to see the light, and many laws have now been instituted that require food manufacturers and/or restaurants to phase out trans fats and, in the meantime, clearly label them. That's good news for you, because you can read the labels on the foods you love to see whether they contain trans fats, saturated fats, and other kinds of fats. So read the label!

You might be wondering about margarine at this point. Traditional margarine is made out of trans fat. It's chemically manipulated and, in my opinion, disgusting. I think it's like eating plastic. Today there are some trans-fat-free margarines, and some are even made with olive oil. These can be okay if you really need to have a buttery schmear on your toast, but personally, I think small amounts of real dairy butter are the superior choice. Your body understands what butter is because it's a real whole food. Unless you absolutely shun animal products (the vegans I know are big fans of Earth Balance, one of the best margarine choices if you want to go there), I strongly suggest sticking with olive oil and other healthy plant sources of fat instead of butter—and occasionally using the real dairy stuff as a treat.

The good news is that some fat is actually *good news*. Fats from plant sources and fish tend to have a positive effect on your health, keeping arteries soft and flexible. In fact, plant fats and fish oil have all kinds of positive effects. They make your skin soft and your hair shiny, and some studies suggest they even improve your mood. Say farewell to PMS, girls!

The good stuff is easy to find and makes your meals more filling and satisfying. So just say no to trans fats and welcome healthy fats that improve your cholesterol and help your heart.

These oils include:

* Olive oil
* Flaxseed oil
* Canola oil

* Fish oil
* Nut oil

Other foods that supply your body with healthy oils include these gems:

* Avocado
* Salmon (and other cold-water fish, like sardines)
* Nuts and seeds (such as hemp seeds, pine nuts, almonds, hazelnuts, sunflower seeds, pumpkin seeds, and even peanuts, which are actually a legume)

Fat still has calories, and too much of any kind of fat isn't good for anyone (just as too much of anything isn't good—moderation, my dear, moderation in all things!). But if you cut the bad fat and add the good fat, I promise you'll start to see some dramatic changes.

So eat your fat. Love it. Drizzle olive oil on toast (add a sprinkle of sea salt—delicious!). Eat more roasted salmon and sushi. Have a handful of nuts for a snack instead of a handful of chips or cookies. Cook with canola oil. And when the occasion warrants it, enjoy a little bit of real, organic, fresh dairy butter. Because you deserve it.

The Ultimate Snack

WHEN I CRAVE salt *and* fat *and* sweet, I've discovered the perfect snack: apples and peanut butter. I've been eating creamy peanut butter on Macintosh apple slices since I was a kid. This was my favorite after-school snack in the fall. I went on to eat them in my college dorm during late-night study sessions, when I was newly married and my husband was out of town (the perfect snacky dinner), and now I serve them on playdates, as a substantial snack for hungry little boys (those without nut allergies, of course). Apples have fiber and juicy sweetness, while peanut butter has protein and the kind of fat that makes you feel full and satisfied and humming with happiness. Snacks in a box? Who needs 'em? Pass me another apple and that jar of peanut butter, please. Want some?

SWEET NOTHINGS

Picture this: A seven-year-old blond girl sits at a kitchen table watching her grandma make her special oatmeal for breakfast. Grandma pours the creamy porridge in a big bowl. The steam rises. She slides it in front of the wide-eyed little girl, who carefully pours on a bit of warm milk and then dips her tiny spoon in the bowl of sparkly sugar once, twice. The little girl (okay, I admit, it's me) slowly stirs the sugar and milk into the oatmeal. The first bite is like heaven: sweet, substantial, satisfying, warm, a veritable *symbol* of Grandma. Ah, it makes me feel good just to remember it.

Sugar is just so darned . . . *pretty*. All crystalline and glittery and snow-white. How could something so good be so bad for you? It took me a long time to accept that sugar might not be okay in any amount. I've always been a sugar fiend, so when I learned about the negative effects sugar can have on the body, I was distraught. How could it be? Sugar, bad? Oh, please say it isn't so!

But it is so, I'm afraid, at least when you're talking about the snow-white stuff. According to the National Cancer Institute, most women consume about eighteen teaspoons of sugar a day, and if you drink a lot of regular soda, you can boost those numbers way up, baby. It's not that a little sugar is going to hurt anyone, but the problem with processed sugar—most widely available in the form of white sugar and high-fructose corn syrup, which you will find, if you read the label, is in almost every processed food on the planet—is that it's addictive. You eat a little, and you want more. And more. And more. Too much sugar wreaks havoc on your insulin levels and can tip you right into a lifelong battle with diabetes. Real Moms who want to avoid disease and illness and low energy and excess weight have to get a handle on their sugar addiction. There's just no way around it.

When I first began my quest for a cleaner, healthier way of life, one of the first changes I made was to get rid of white sugar and high-fructose corn syrup. I refused to eat it. I decided to get it O-U-T of my house. I was shocked to find it in bread, mayonnaise, cereals, sauce, ketchup, crackers, soup. All that stuff went straight into the trash.

Sometimes it was disguised, wearing funny names like a fake mustache and glasses—dextrose, sucrose, maltose. But I knew better. It was all sugar.

And what about America's new favorite villain, high-fructose corn syrup, ominously referred to in the media these days as HFCS? (Doesn't it sound like some code for a government conspiracy or a secret military operation? "White dove, white dove, alert, alert, HFCS is on the move; the mission has been compromised!")

Like trans fats, high-fructose corn syrup is a chemically derived pseudofood ingredient. The glucose in cornstarch is converted to fructose, making a kind of Franken-sugar hybrid of fructose and glucose that doesn't decay (since it's fake) and can extend the shelf life of processed foods, from sodas to snack cakes, for oh, let's say *decades*? Does anyone want a Twinkie? They were freshly baked in 1990! Okay, perhaps I exaggerate, but you get my point. HFCS as well as trans fats allow us to eat *old food*. Oh, boy. My favorite.

As for health, research is conflicting, although one always has to wonder who is paying for the studies that say these fake foods are just fine. Some studies do show an association between HFCS ingestion and obesity, particularly childhood obesity, as well as insulin resistance and diabetes.

Personally, I'd rather not wait around for the science to tell me that fake food is quite definitely proven to be bad for my health and the health of my children. As a Real Mom, you need to make food choices that are going to help you feel good, look good, and stay healthy. If you ask me, any food containing HFCS does not qualify. I strongly encourage you to rid your family's diet of HFCS from today onward. Just look at those labels and raid that pantry.

After I did this in my own kitchen, however, what was I left with? A barren wasteland of a diet with no sweetness to brighten my day? Let me tell you, I wasted no time finding acceptable substitutes for my "fix."

Sweet isn't bad. Processed sugar is bad. You don't have to give up your sweetness. I discovered many healthy whole-food alternatives to sugar, and I never looked back—natural sweeteners that are relatively unprocessed, and full of micronutrients that are a mere fond memory for your frenemy white sugar.

When I gave up processed sugar, I dropped pounds without even trying, because natural sugars are more satisfying. Those micronutrients tell your body you actually ate something, so natural sugars don't typically trigger an obsessive need for more. Here's what I now eat instead of sugar:

* **FRUIT:** You've probably eaten too many cookies, but have you ever been compelled to eat too many apples?
* **AGAVE NECTAR:** This syrup from the blue agave cactus is the stuff they distill to make tequila. It tastes a bit like honey, but mellower and milder. Use it as you would use honey or maple syrup. Agave nectar has only a slight impact on your blood sugar—nothing compared to the white stuff.
* **HONEY:** This bee-derived sweetener gives you a quick energy boost but contains protein, vitamins, and minerals, unlike white sugar. It's a whole food, so your body knows what to do with it. You may also be able to buy local honey made from local bees and local flowers, which is good for your local economy and the environment.
* **MAPLE SYRUP, BROWN-RICE SYRUP, BARLEY MALT, SORGHUM, AND MOLASSES:** These natural sweeteners are good for baking or drizzling on your pancakes or Grandma's oatmeal. They are very sweet, like sugar, so don't overdo it. The nutrients make these a superior choice to sugar.
* **MAPLE SUGAR, DATE SUGAR, AND SUCANAT:** Granulated sweeteners rich with micronutrients. (Sucanat is nonrefined granulated sugarcane juice.)
* **STEVIA:** A sweet herb with zero calories, stevia is an excellent alternative to chemically derived artificial sweeteners. Stevia has been in the press a lot lately as a natural alternative to sugar. I love it. It's actually a sweet herb that is minimally processed into a powder that is about fifteen times as sweet as sugar, so you don't need nearly as much, and it has virtually no calories. Some people think that it can have a bitter aftertaste if you use too much; I find that just a little sprinkle when I need a shot of sweetness is pleasant and perfect. You may or may not like stevia, but I hope you will try it. It won't play games with your insulin levels, but it will satisfy your sweet tooth.

Just in Case You Weren't Listening
(or Are Still in Denial)...

SO, YOU'RE THINKING that you're just fine, you with your can of diet soda, and I can just keep my fancy-schmancy brown-rice syrups and agave nectars and whatnot because your diet drink has no calories?

Now, wait one minute. I think it's been, what . . . several pages since I've ranted about artificial sweetener? No time like the present to do it again.

Just in case you're still considering a flirtation with the nasty chemical brews known as diet drinks, let me remind you that you are *drinking chemicals*. Experimental chemicals, at that. I've seen so much convincing evidence that artificial sweeteners can do horrible things to your health that I refuse to touch them. I would never allow my kids to touch them.

Plus, a University of Texas Health Science Center survey in 2005 found that people who drink diet soft drinks may actually gain weight; in that study, for every can of diet soda people consumed each day, there was a 41 percent increased risk of being overweight. So . . . you want to drink something that could make you sick and increase your risk of being fat? Because it has no calories?

I'm no radical, I swear. I'm just a regular Real Mom who is fiercely protective of her kids. Just forget the soda. Move on, children. It's killing your brains, whether it's artificially sweetened or swimming with HFCS. And Real Moms? Seriously. Just say no.

You'll notice I don't suggest you quit eating sweetener altogether. Some people advocate this. They say you don't need sweets, and physically, they're right; it's just that life is more fun with some sweet stuff in it. But if you're ready to go without, good for you. Just be prepared: Going cold turkey off of sugar can result in some withdrawal symptoms, such as headaches and irritability. However, if you want to go for it, you have my blessing. Just remember to eat something every three to four hours, so you avoid a blood sugar drop that can make you crave sweets.

But if you like your life with a little sugar, I totally get it. Go ahead. Dabble in the sweet stuff, but purge the sweet nothings from your life—you'll look and feel better almost immediately!

DO FIVE THINGS

I hope I've inspired you to give your dysfunctional dietary friends a strict talking-to, to ditch their trashier personas and replace them with a better class of deliciousness. Consider it an intervention. Here's what I want you to do this week:

1. GIVE PROCESSED FOOD THE BOOT AND UPGRADE YOUR TABLE SALT. THE MORE INTENSE FLAVORS IN GOURMET SALTS HELP YOU USE LESS.

Just get into those cupboards and purge. If you can't stand to throw out all the processed food (and in these frugal days, who can?), use these criteria. Throw it out if it has:

* Over 200 milligrams of sodium per serving
* Any trans fats (any ingredients with the words *hydroge-nated* or *partially hydrogenated*)
* Any high-fructose corn syrup
* Any processed sugar (might appear as a chemical name ending in *-ose*, such as glucose, maltose, or fructose—especially check your beverages!)
* Any artificial sweetener

Then (am I cheating; is this two things to do?) throw out the processed table salt and get some unrefined sea salt and, as the mood strikes you, splurge on the occasional gourmet salt—pink, gray, red, black, smoked, whatever. It's a whole new world out there, salt lovers. Get picky and you'll be richly rewarded.

2. BUY THREE NEW HERBS OR SPICES AND START USING THEM ON YOUR FOOD.

This week, live on the edge. Find three new seasonings or herbs and experiment with them this week. Get to know how they taste. Decide whether you like them or not. Paprika? Oregano? Curry powder? Sage? Coriander? Tarragon? Fenugreek? Herbs gone wild!

3. BANISH EVIL TRANS FATS FROM YOUR HOME FOR GOOD.

Throw the bums out! Trade all trans fat products for those containing olive oil, canola oil, nut oils, or real butter. Always keep a big bottle of good extra virgin olive oil handy.

Make your own simple salad dressing using olive oil and a splash of red wine vinegar or balsamic vinegar or citrus juice (two parts oil to one part vinegar or juice) and a dash of good salt and freshly ground black pepper. (Bonus points for homemade: the bottled stuff usually contains high-fructose corn syrup!) Sauté with good oils, or use cooking spray or a splash of chicken broth. If you've really already thrown out all the trans fats from your pantry, then this one will be easy.

4. GET RID OF SWEET NOTHINGS LIKE WHITE SUGAR, HIGH-FRUCTOSE CORN SYRUP, AND ARTIFICIAL SWEETENER.

Sugar? You don't need no stinkin' sugar. Explore the charms of natural sweeteners this week. If these are new to you, start with the mildest, agave nectar, and start to feel the magic: freedom from sugar addiction!

5. DRINK SIX GLASSES OF FRESH, PURE WATER EVERY DAY.

I'm going to up your intake yet again, girlfriends, and here's why: When you banish the toxic stuff from your life, your body amps up the cleansing process, and you'll need lots of fresh, pure water to help wash that junk out of your system. Just keep swilling it, Real Moms. I know what I'm talking about. In a week, you're going to feel a whole new level of clean energy.

I want to end with an important note about water bottles. I'm known in some circles as the "Green Mom" because I often talk about and write about how to live a more ecofriendly life without being too extreme. Therefore, wearing that particular hat, I would be remiss if I didn't say that plastic water bottles are one of the largest contributors to landfill trash. Even if you recycle the plastic, you are still contributing to the solid-waste problem more than if you drink your water out of a sturdy, reusable, nontoxic water bottle that you wash every day. Or you could try an actual glass.

Maybe it's slightly more trouble to fill up and wash out a water bottle that you have to tote with you all the time, but really, everybody is doing it, and you can buy cute stainless-steel ones with funky designs (stay away from plastic water bottles unless they are free of BPA, a nasty chemical often used in plastics—more about that later). Besides, is it that much trouble compared to the trouble the world will face when it's all filled up with trash and we have to start shooting our junk out into space? I got used to carrying my own water bottle, and I'm pretty sure you can too, especially if you have any motivation to keep the world nice and tidy and actually functional for your kids' future use.

WEEK FOUR:

Tame the Food-cravings Dragon

THIS WEEK, DO FIVE THINGS:

1. Eat breakfast every day, consisting of complex carbs and some protein, and add a high-quality vitamin/mineral supplement to your routine every morning, taken just before eating breakfast.

2. Whenever a craving strikes, have a glass of water and eat something from the energy snacks list on page 69 before you do anything rash. After eating, wait twenty minutes. Then, if you are still having your craving, portion it out and enjoy it.

3. Drink seven glasses of fresh, pure water every day.

4. Make a list of the dysfunctional foods you crave. Next to each one, make a list of upgraded choices for every dysfunctional food you tend to crave. Replace the bad stuff with ingredients to make the good stuff and then dig in. (I'll show you how.)

5. Not all cravings are for the bad stuff. Think of your absolute favorite life-enhancing, pleasurable, sexy foods you sometimes crave. Go out and buy three of them. When you need an indulgence, go for one of these. Or develop a new healthy obsession and let yourself crave it and enjoy it.

DID I EVER tell you I'm psychic? I am; just watch. I know what you're thinking right now. Okay, just close your eyes and concentrate very hard. I will too. I'll put my hands to my temples and hum mystically.

You are thinking of . . . chocolate!

Hmm, maybe I'm projecting. Because *I'm* thinking of chocolate. I think of chocolate a *lot*. And I'm not ashamed! However, as you may already know, food cravings can be pretty powerful. They can hijack your brain and make you do things you never would have done if you were thinking straight, like eat the entire box of cookies or the whole bag of chips. *Wait . . . wasn't this bag of chips full a few minutes ago? Where did they all go? (Delicate burp.)*

Cravings can feel like an addiction, like a monkey on your back, like a dragon that constantly terrorizes you. We all think about our favorite foods sometimes, relishing the memory, looking forward to our next indulgence, but out-of-control cravings are different. They prompt you to eat those foods, the ones that should be a once-in-a-while indulgence, *all the time.*

It's no way to live, Real Moms. But flex your biceps and make a fist and take a Rosie-the-Riveter stance with me right now—we can kick those cravings in the behind. We can slay that dragon. *We can do it!*

THE ANATOMY OF A FOOD CRAVING

They say you should keep your friends close and your enemies closer. They say knowledge is power. So let's delve into this whole cravings thing and take it apart and see what we've got. When you understand what's going on, you can begin to deal more rationally with the dragon.

People have a lot of different ideas about cravings. Some people think cravings are a sign of weakness, that cravings must be beaten into submission, that a craving should never be indulged, and if it is, it is a sign that you have no willpower and might as well just give up and eat anything and everything that crosses your path.

Others say that cravings are the body's wise signal that you need some kind of nutrient, and even if your mind interprets, "I need energy," as, "I need Milk Duds," a valid biological requirement exists at the heart of the craving.

I say the truth is somewhere in the middle.

The human body *is* amazing; it's true. Just think about it for a minute. It knows when to go to sleep, to wake up, to go to the bathroom. It knows exactly how to maintain an internal temperature of 98.6 degrees, and it jacks up the heat only when it's got an infection to kill. It beats its own heart, distributes its blood, closes its eyes in response to hazards, sends quick energy to its muscles when it senses the need to react quickly; it breathes, and it can even reproduce. Pretty incredible. It's more miraculous, skilled, and complicated than the world's most advanced supercomputer.

So it seems like there must be *something* to a craving. And there is. One of the things your body does, all on its own, is to try to maintain the sugar level in your blood at a constant rate. When you haven't eaten anything in a while, your blood sugar level starts to drop. In response, your body sends signals to your brain that say, *Eat something!* If you've gone a really long time without eating, your body sends a more urgent signal: *Eat something quick! And make it full of energy, because I'm running on empty!*

And what's the most easily available source of quick energy? Simple carbs and sugar. That's right—chocolate, candy, potato chips, French fries, cookies, crackers, movie popcorn. . . .

There is nothing wrong with carbohydrates. They appear everywhere in the foods nature provides us—in fruits, vegetables, and whole grains. They are made up of long chains of sugars bound up in fiber. When you eat these foods, your body slowly breaks down the fiber in order to get to the sugars, which are then absorbed into your bloodstream gradually.

The key word is *gradually*. If you respond to this so-called biological emergency by eating too many simple carbs and sugars, especially without any fiber, your blood sugar goes too high too fast, like that roller coaster you vowed never to go on again. Insulin, a hormone secreted by your poor, put-upon pancreas, is released in response to blood sugar to help your body use the sugars for energy, but too much blood sugar can trigger too much insulin, which results in a massive drop in blood sugar. That roller coaster tips downward into a free fall, and then guess what? Your blood sugar plummets and you're starving all over again, even though you just ate a whole box of cookies.

This is why starting your day with a doughnut can keep you hungry all day long, while starting your day with whole grains and some protein, like steel-cut oats with milk, or whole-grain toast with peanut butter, will keep you on a more even keel.

When you indulge too frequently in simple carbs, this radical blood sugar game can wreak havoc on your body. It can even cause type 2 diabetes. If you have this condition (or its precursor, insulin resistance), your body gets so numbed by the blood-sugar-versus-insulin war that it stops responding well to insulin. That can tip you into some seriously debilitating and potentially deadly health consequences.

So you can see where those cravings could lead . . . and it's not somewhere you want to go. If you are already there, you know what I mean.

The good news is that even if you are edging towards insulin resistance or type 2 diabetes, you can head back in the other direction all on your own steam. And if you aren't there, or aren't there yet, you never have to go that way.

But you are going to have to do something about that dragon.

EATING FOR ENERGY

When you give in to a craving with a poor choice, you risk sapping your energy for the rest of the day. Sometimes I think of my energy level as if it's a bottle of laundry detergent. When you get to the end of the bottle and realize you have only a little bit left, you can get frantic about getting just *one more load out of that bottle*! I've been known to have a couple of upside-down laundry detergent bottles in my laundry room, propped in the strangest ways, dripping out the last precious drops. Do you try to squeeze the last few drops from yourself when you are exhausted and feel like you can barely take another step or think another productive thought? I hear that.

When you are "out of blood sugar," don't settle for a quick fix that will tide you over for half an hour, or "one more load of laundry." Eat the right kind of snack and you'll set yourself back up with a full bottle of detergent, so to speak. For example, if I eat a bagel, I get a quick rush of energy, and then I'm exhausted. But if I eat a bowl of quinoa and vegetables, I'm replenished for hours.

There is one very simple way to get control of your blood sugar: Every time you eat, include some protein (meat, fish, chicken, nuts, seeds, protein powdered drink or bar, or eggs), complex carbs (any form of grain that is not processed and has its fiber intact, such as whole grains, oats, quinoa, brown rice), and fiber (found in whole fruit, vegetables, and the whole grains listed above). Even if it's just a little, if you include all three components (protein, complex carbs, and fiber) in every meal and snack, your blood sugar is much more likely to stay steady. Including protein, complex carbs, and fiber *every time you eat* will change your life, I swear. No more chips-and-a-soda snacks for you, missy. Is that momentary mind-numbing pleasure worth an entire day of torturous cravings and that dead-tired feeling of total exhaustion? I didn't think so.

Some foods simply sap your energy. These include too much of any of the following:

* Caffeine
* Alcohol
* Fatty protein
* Any food containing processed sugar and/or white flour

I'm not saying you can't eat these things, but if you do choose to eat them, limit the amount or you'll pay the price.

Other foods give you more energy than you had before you ate them. Obviously, those are the foods you want to choose for your snacks, and to buck those cravings for the bad stuff that will make you feel even worse.

But what to eat? I'm at your service. This list of energy foods can be your go-to snack list. Whenever you feel a craving—*whenever you feel a craving!*—choose something from this list first. I predict you'll nip that gastronomic desperation in the bud.

Energy Snacks

- ¼ cup almonds, walnuts, peanuts, or mixed nuts and a handful of grapes
- Half a tuna fish sandwich on whole-grain bread
- Peach, pear, or apple with 1 ounce of cheese or 1 tablespoon of peanut butter
- ½ cup cooked whole grains with ¼ cup beans (examples: brown rice and red beans, polenta and black beans, bulgur and white beans—make ahead and keep in the refrigerator to snack on all week)
- 1 cup of cooked quinoa with a handful of sautéed veggies
- ½ cup cooked oatmeal with 1 tablespoon chopped walnuts and regular or soy milk
- ½ cup hummus with 6 baby carrots
- Whole-grain toast with tomato slice and avocado slice (and a dash of sea salt)
- 1 cup leafy greens (like kale, Swiss chard, or collard greens), chopped and quickly sautéed in 1 teaspoon olive oil with ½ cup extra-firm tofu cubes and 1 clove garlic. Season with salt and pepper.
- Whole-grain toast with 1 tablespoon sesame butter and 1 teaspoon of molasses drizzled on top, sprinkled with a teaspoon of wheat germ or ground flaxseed
- Bowl of leafy greens and any chopped raw vegetables, tossed with 1 tablespoon each olive oil, lemon juice, and grated cheese
- Smoothie made with ½ cup yogurt, 1 cup fresh or frozen fruit, 1 tablespoon ground flaxseed, 1 scoop protein powder, and a splash of fresh juice or water to blend. If you are having a chocolate craving, add a dash of cinnamon and 1 teaspoon cocoa powder or raw cacao.

THE OTHER SIDE OF CRAVINGS

Unfortunately, out-of-whack blood sugar isn't the whole story.

Cravings have a lot to do with blood sugar levels, but they also have something to do with another culprit, one that's clever at disguising its influence. Yes, brain, I'm talking to you. Your brain gets *used to* things. It likes to form habits. It responds well to pleasure and it doesn't respond so well to pain, stress, and unpleasant feelings.

Sometimes, when your brain experiences an unpleasant thought or feeling, it tries to distract itself by making you think of food. *I'm bored. Let's eat! I'm sad. Let's eat! I'm nervous. Let's eat! I have way too much to do today. I know—let's eat!*

Many Real Moms know all about emotional eating, and eating in response to stress, boredom, or simply out of habit (you turn on the TV and your brain flips a switch: *Let's eat!*), but knowing that you are in the throes of emotional eating doesn't do all that much to stop the momentum.

So what's a Real Mom to make of this complex and interesting process behind what seems to be a pretty basic craving for a Hershey bar or a sack of fries? Luckily for us all, I have some answers. When I was studying at the Institute for Integrative Nutrition, I learned that there are eight primary causes for cravings:

1. **DEHYDRATION.** When you are low on water, your body can get confused and send a signal to hydrate that your brain interprets as a signal to eat. Whenever you get a craving, *always drink a glass of water first.*

2. **LACK OF LIFE FULFILLMENT.** When you think you want a cookie, you might really want more or less mental or emotional stimulation. Being dissatisfied with a relationship, being too stressed about work or family problems, being bored, feeling uninspired by your job, lacking a spiritual component to your life . . . all can lead to a feeling of hunger. And it *is* hunger, but not for food. Later in this book, I'll talk more about how to reduce stress and enrich your life in other ways that can

help reduce cravings, but for now, just be aware that your cravings might actually be for something that has nothing to do with that cookie.

3. **YIN/YANG IMBALANCE.** Pardon me while I get all Far East for a minute, but the concept of yin (expansive, light, assertive) and yang (contractive, dark, receptive) as balancing forces in all aspects of life is an ancient one that can be helpful in recognizing a lack of balance in contemporary life. Striving for a yin/yang balance in everything you do can help you feel calmer and more centered. Also, according to some theories (including macrobiotics), food exists on a scale from yin to yang, with sugar and raw food on the far yin end and meat and cooked food on the far yang end. If you eat strictly from one side, you can get out of balance and crave things from the other side of the spectrum. So if you are craving meat and warm cooked food because you've been eating too much sugar and cold raw food, or vice versa, then go ahead and get back into balance. Just do it wisely—not with a cheeseburger (for more yang) or a slab of cake (for more yin) but with, let's just say, a warm bowl of chicken soup (for more yang) or a fresh, crisp salad of organic vegetables (for more yin).

4. **SECURITY.** Your brain enjoys regularity and familiarity, and that can be a source of cravings, especially when you are feeling insecure or anxious about something new. Your brain turns to something familiar, like something you just ate yesterday when you were feeling good, or something you loved as a child. There is nothing wrong with seeking comfort from food, as long as you discover comfort from a healthy food. Look for a healthy version of the familiar food you crave and you'll get the stabilizing effect without compromising your health.

5. **SEASONAL.** If you get really good at listening to your body and you tend to eat in harmony with the seasons (always a good idea), you may notice your body craving the foods that are in season, like leafy greens in spring,

fruit and juicy vegetables in the summer, richer vegetables in the fall, and warm soups and fattier foods in the winter. Cravings may also arise in association with your memories of certain holidays—turkey and pumpkin pie on Thanksgiving, sweets during the winter holidays, barbecue on Independence Day. These are all fine cravings if you satisfy them with nutritious foods.

6. **LACK OF NUTRIENTS.** Sometimes a craving really is a sign of a nutritional deficiency. You may crave salt if you are dehydrated or are missing some mineral. You may crave sweets if you are lacking some vitamins that you could get from a juicy, sweet piece of fruit. To cover your bases, take a high-quality vitamin and mineral supplement.

7. **HORMONAL.** Hear ye, hear ye, PMS-ers, pregnant girlfriends, postpartum new mamas, and perimenopausal sisters—your hormones are playing tricks on you! Hormone fluctuations during these womanly events can cause strange cravings because of low serotonin levels, which can trigger an intense desire for carbohydrates. Easy does it, because too dramatic a response can make your uncomfortable physical symptoms worse.

8. **DEVOLUTION.** Just like that philosophy professor or physics major you had a crush on in college, brains are just so . . . *inscrutable*. Sometimes when things are going really well, your brain can decide that things are going *too* well and you can begin to sabotage yourself, craving things that will throw your blood sugar out of whack and plunge you into feeling bad again. Silly, but it happens. Just like that crush.

Knowing the source of your cravings is the first step to conquering them, but it's not enough in itself. In order to lasso the dragon and take charge of your food choices, you have to get your blood sugar under control, and then you have to get your *brain* under control. It's a big job, but nothing a Real Mom can't handle. When you establish new habits, new triggers, and healthier choices for your cravings, you'll step into the light and never look back. Because that dragon is *toast*.

DO FIVE THINGS

Are you ready to conquer the dragon? All you have to do this week is five simple things that will help you get your cravings under your thumb. No more monkey on your back. No more dragon breathing down your neck. Just fabulous you, deciding with a rational mind exactly what you *really* want to eat.

1. EAT BREAKFAST EVERY DAY, CONSISTING OF COMPLEX CARBS AND SOME PROTEIN, AND ADD A HIGH-QUALITY VITAMIN/MINERAL SUPPLEMENT TO YOUR ROUTINE EVERY MORNING, TAKEN JUST BEFORE EATING BREAKFAST.

Start every day this week right, with your dragon-slaying sword made of protein and complex carbs. Whatever you choose—eggs and whole-grain toast, oatmeal with walnuts and milk, yogurt with fruit and nuts, a green smoothie with protein powder, or something else you love—just keep the sugar out and the fiber and protein in. Add a multivitamin/mineral supplement to guard against any nutritional deficiencies that could be triggering cravings. Take it with breakfast, for best absorption. That dragon won't stand a chance.

2. WHENEVER A CRAVING STRIKES, HAVE A GLASS OF WATER AND EAT SOMETHING FROM THE ENERGY SNACKS LIST ON PAGE 69 BEFORE YOU DO ANYTHING RASH. AFTER EATING, WAIT TWENTY MINUTES. THEN, IF YOU STILL HAVE YOUR CRAVING, PORTION IT OUT AND ENJOY IT.

Remember that dehydration can cause cravings, so always have water first, then a snack from your trusty energy snacks list. Whenever you do this, you are training your body to handle cravings properly, not dysfunctionally. Then, if the craving remains, have a little bit of what you really want, even if it's candy or potato chips. One serving isn't going to hurt you. However, I'm guessing that your energy snack will slay that dragon and you'll forget all about that snack you thought you wanted.

3. DRINK SEVEN GLASSES OF FRESH, PURE WATER EVERY DAY.

See above note about dehydration. Your water is more important than ever this week, so just keep going—I'm so proud of how you are staying hydrated and healthy! This week, you might try slicing some lemons, limes, or oranges and floating a few slices in your water glass or in a pitcher of water you keep in your refrigerator. Or try slices of cucumber for an extra-refreshing glass of the wet stuff. Always keep a glass on your nightstand, and have a swig every morning, first thing (it's good for your teeth too!).

And if you want to get really "green," do what I do—use that leftover water on your nightstand to brush your teeth in the morning. Why waste more water when you've got some sitting right there? Are you laughing at me? Am I too extreme? I don't think so! We take for granted how precious water is. I don't like to waste a drop.

4. MAKE A LIST OF THE DYSFUNCTIONAL FOODS YOU CRAVE. NEXT TO EACH ONE, MAKE A LIST OF UPGRADED CHOICES FOR EACH ONE—HOW CAN YOU MAKE BETTER COOKIES, PIZZA, NACHOS, SODA, OR PASTA? REPLACE THE BAD STUFF WITH INGREDIENTS TO MAKE THE GOOD STUFF AND THEN DIG IN.

When I think of the word *dysfunctional*, I think of problems, issues, baggage. When I think of dysfunctional foods, I see them in the same way—as foods that create problems, issues, and excess baggage (on your hips, thighs, upper arms, rear). Bad habits are tough to kick, but if you can replace those foods that make you go weak in the knees with something close but more nutritious, you won't feel so deprived.

This week, make a list of your food weaknesses—the foods that make you crazy with desire. Then think about how you might still be able to enjoy those foods in a healthier way—baked chips and low-fat cheese nachos instead of the full-fat version? Veggie pizza instead of sausage? A strict one-cookie policy?

I crave plenty of not-so-nutritious foods, but I've learned how to make little changes in my habits like these, so I'm nourishing myself, not hurting myself, when cravings strike. To get you started on your list, I'll show you mine:

* **MOVIE POPCORN.** I confessed my weakness in chapter three. I've discovered that if I have just a salad for dinner, I absolutely can't pass up the popcorn at the movies. However, if I eat something salty and buttery for dinner—something small, like an ear of corn or a baked potato with salt and butter—then I'm not quite so tempted. I just tell myself, *You already had some corn. You don't need any more!*

Instead, I go for something sweet. Amazingly, a small box of candy has hundreds fewer calories and fat grams than a movie popcorn, so it's actually a better choice. And I've learned to never, ever go to the movies hungry, because I know I'll regret it later.

* **BROWNIES.** Me + Chocolate = True Love 4Ever! I would wash your car for a plate of brownies with whipped cream, I swear.

But brownies can be fat bombs and sugar land mines. My solution is to make raw brownies! No, it's not raw brownie batter; it's a fantastic and nutritious concoction of dried fruit, nuts, and chocolate that launches me straight to heaven. I always keep the following ingredients on hand so I can whip up these raw brownies whenever a craving strikes:

> 3 cups raw walnut halves
> 16 pitted dates
> 2/3 cup raw cacao powder (or 1/2 cup cocoa powder)
> 1/4 cup raw cacao nibs (or mini chocolate chips)
> 1/4 cup raisins, dried cherries, or dried cranberries.

Put each ingredient in the food processor, in order, processing each addition for about eight pulses. Press into an 8"x 8" ungreased pan and refrigerate for at least 30 minutes. Cut into 12 squares and then scoop one out for yourself and savor every sweet, chocolaty, heavenly nibble. (You will only need a tiny piece.)

* **MILE-HIGH PLATE OF PASTA.** Back when I used to run marathons, one of my favorite parts of the experience was the postrun meal. I loved the runner's high after a swift ten-miler, but nothing compared to the reward of a huge plate of angel hair pasta with red sauce and a tender juicy meatball on top after a long race. But white pasta is like eating

a plate of sugar—it all turns into glucose in your body. I was so fixated on the taste, however, that I couldn't even think about saying no.

Today, I still don't say no to pasta, but I've found it pays to keep my portions smaller. I never eat more than one cup of cooked pasta in a meal, and I usually try to keep it to half a cup.

I've also upgraded my pasta choice. Now I use Dreamfields pasta, because it has a low glycemic index (it doesn't skyrocket your blood sugar). I also like some of the other higher-protein pastas on the market, like those produced by Dr. Barry Sears at zonediet.com. Another solution in a pinch: brown rice with a drizzle of marinara sauce and a meatball. I still get the satisfaction, without the blood sugar crash and the extra layer of padding on my thighs.

* **WHIPPED CREAM.** This is one of those childhood obsessions. When I was in grade school, my aunt used to spray whipped topping directly into my mouth, while I thanked the whipped cream gods for their bountiful blessings. When I would close my mouth, the creamy white fluff would inevitably overflow. If I was quick enough, I'd catch the excess with my hands and shovel it back in, not wanting to miss a single fluffy molecule of pure whipped pleasure. I still don't think a hot-fudge sundae is worth its salted nuts without a whipped cream top-off.

These days I try to control myself, and I don't *usually* actually squirt the whipped topping directly into my piehole, but I do still enjoy whipped cream's whimsical qualities, on very special occasions. It's no longer an every-weekend kind of affair.

Real whipped cream isn't hard to make. You buy a carton of heavy cream and whip it up in minutes with your electric beater or (if you've got strong biceps) a wire whisk and your own power. However, there are easier options—just read the label! Some brands of spray whipped cream are pretty pure, mostly just cream and sugar, as you might make at home. If you prefer the kind in the tub, avoid those with high-fructose corn syrup and trans fats. One option I like, when I'm in that kind of mood, is Truwhip, a mostly nondairy whipped topping without the HFCS and trans fats of more popular brands.

* **BANANA LAFFY TAFFY.** Am I ridiculous? I think not! Why shouldn't I love the chewy, stretchy, banana-y stuff? Sure, it's artificially flavored. It's artificially colored. It's not nutritious in any way. But c'mon . . . it's *Laffy Taffy*! I have been known to compete with the six-year-olds when the parade float riders throw candy into the crowd on the Fourth of July. They can keep their Tootsie Rolls and licorice whips, but I'm diving into the street for that Laffy Taffy. I'm just saying.

However, I have noticed, now that I'm no longer twelve, that I don't always digest candy very well. Whatever it is, I've decided that most of the time I don't need to eat it, but on the Fourth of July, I can allow myself a couple of pieces— just enough to get that Laffy Taffy experience without the candy hangover. On any other day, I'll satisfy my craving with a much more nutritious banana smoothie made with chocolate almond milk and a dash of agave nectar.

* **KETTLE CHIPS.** When I get that salty itch, chips take the cake. I can go for weeks, even months, without craving them, but when I get the chip urge, get out of my way. I especially love the extraauthoritative crunch of handmade kettle chips. Kettle chips actually sound wholesome, don't you think? After all, they're cooked in a *kettle*. My grandmother cooked food in a kettle, and it was always wholesome. One of the reasons I like kettle chips is because they are cooked by hand in small batches and only kissed with a little salt. One serving, about thirteen chips, has 9 grams of fat, 16 grams of carbs, and 2 grams of protein. That's not so bad for an occasional indulgence. I feel better choosing the organic kind, because I know they won't contain any pesticides or other chemical residue. My compromise is to never let myself eat them out of the bag. I portion out one serving and have them only every so often, when I really, really want them. Then it's totally worth the splurge.

5. NOT ALL CRAVINGS ARE FOR THE BAD STUFF. THINK OF YOUR ABSOLUTE FAVORITE LIFE-ENHANCING, PLEASURABLE, SEXY FOODS YOU SOMETIMES CRAVE. GO OUT AND BUY THREE OF THEM. WHEN YOU NEED AN INDULGENCE, GO FOR ONE OF THESE. OR DEVELOP A NEW HEALTHY OBSESSION AND LET YOURSELF CRAVE IT AND ENJOY IT.

You aren't all bad. I swear you aren't. I know you feel passionate about some foods that really are excellent nutritional choices that energize you and make you feel amazing. So what's your pleasure? A juicy ripe peach? Peanut butter? Creamy yogurt with blueberries and mini chocolate chips? Spicy chili on a cold day, or a really fresh, crisp, cold salad on a hot day? Raspberry sorbet? Cinnamon-scented coffee? A really good wedge of French Brie?

Maybe you *have* to have a spoonful of cocoa powder in your smoothie every morning because that's *your thing*. Excellent! Are you a sucker for a good fruit salad as long as it's sprinkled with coconut? Do you have aspirations to become a sourdough special-ist? A cheese connoisseur? An organic gardener?

The world of amazing and healthy food is your oyster. (Maybe oysters will be your next new thing!) So why have you been limiting your cravings to a few uninspired junk-food choices? Let yourself go wild in the world of great food and discover a whole new level of gastronomic pleasure.

This week, choose three nutritious foods you absolutely love, and then keep them in your kitchen. Enjoy them at will. Let your-self revel in their deliciousness. Rave about them to your friends. Not sure how to start? Maybe I can inspire you.

In the last few years, I've made a hobby out of my passion for the most vibrant, gorgeous, amazing, fresh plant food. Anyone who knows me knows that my refrigerator has more food in it than my pantry. Aside from a couple of boxes of organic cereal and organic crunchy snacks for the kids, like pretzels, rice chips and corn puffs. I really don't house a lot of canned or boxed foods.

I do, however, *always* have bowls of (in-season) fruits, nuts, seeds, and veggies on hand, like snap peas, mini carrots and celery—especially cut up for the kids to eat when they get home.

One of my favorites is grapefruit. I swoon when my mom tells me she's sent me a box of her hybrid, übersweet grapefruit. They should be illegal, they're so sweet and addictive. I will cut up two and eat them at my computer, or snag one on the way out the door and hide it in my purse for nibbling later in the day. I used to devour grapefruit as a child. I still remember my grandmother's grapefruit spoon, with the teeth at the tip for spooning out the most possible fruit and juice, leaving the scraped-clean hollow yellow shell. I used to love to turn the bare, dry rind, bereft of a single drop of that sweet-sour juice, inside out, just to prove to myself (and any nearby adults I hoped to impress) that I'd eaten every possible bit.

When I was a kid, I sprinkled sugar on top, like most grapefruit rookies. However, as time went by, I found I didn't need it. I felt so grown-up when I graduated from the sugar bowl. And then . . . the first time I ever tasted my mom's hybrid grapefruit, I was in heaven. I had discovered a sacred fruit that no one else (except mom and her sister) had ever tasted. This secret stash makes my trips to Phoenix so special, as my mom and I still walk among her fruit trees, admiring the flowers that will soon produce fruit and, if I'm lucky, are in bloom when I go to visit. If there's a box in the mail headed in my direction, I will wait by the mailbox, mouth watering.

Another fruity favorite of mine is blueberries. I can't get enough of these candylike sweets. In the summertime, I go to the farmers' markets looking for fresh crops, and my kids love them as much as I do. I buy them in bulk and freeze them for a crisp fall day when my smoothie calls for a hint of blue.

And do you mind if I wax poetic for just a moment about cinnamon? Cinnamon is truly a gift from God. It is so magical. The mere scent of it drives me wild. It brings me back to the days when we'd butter our white bread and sprinkle store-bought cinnamon sugar all over it.

Today, I know that it can help lower my cholesterol and regulate my blood sugar, and has an anti-clotting effect. To me, it just tastes great in my hot tea and smoothies or sprinkled on my oatmeal.

And in my reverie, I certainly don't mean to give vegetables the short end of the culinary stick. Because did someone say Brussels sprouts? OMG, I love those little green-headed babies. I know they're good for me, but they could be Laffy Taffy for all I know, I love them so. When combined with a whole-grain rice, Brussels sprouts become an entire meal (as the grain helps complete the relatively high protein in the sprouts), and they have about 3 to 5 grams of fiber per cup, keeping things moving in the digestive system. Sauté them with onions and a hint of garlic and you'll have me at "Hello, would you like some Brussels sprouts?"

I'll end with just a little bit of beefy reverie. Steak filet is such a ladylike steak. I know not all Real Moms are red-meat eaters, but I eat it about once a week or so, for variety and balance and just because I love a really good steak. As you may have guessed, I always choose organic meat, steering clear of anything containing hormone or antibiotic residue. But I don't steer clear of beef—it's one of the building blocks of lean muscle mass and a great source of vitamin B12, supporting a healthy nervous system, and carnitine, which is essential for a healthy heart.

I love cooking my steaks on the grill (avoid charring the outside of the beef, as burned meat may contain carcinogenic compounds). I cook it slowly over medium heat. In the winter I'll broil it, or cook it in the oven, marinated in Dijon mustard, olive oil, soy sauce, Worcestershire sauce, and black pepper, until medium rare, just like my grandmother always did.

Ah, food, glorious food. When you embrace real, whole foods from nature and minimize the junk, that dragon tames down into quite a nice little house pet that can tempt you into the occasional indulgence, but which is perfectly house-trained and under your control at all times. That's what smart eating can do to your cravings—tame them, for your own enjoyment. Because food should give you pleasure, never pain.

WEEK FIVE:

Get Naked with Raw Foods

THIS WEEK, DO FIVE THINGS:

1. Add something raw to every breakfast.
2. Add something raw to every lunch.
3. Add something raw to every dinner.
4. Keep three different raw snacks you really like in your kitchen at all times. Actually snack on them!
5. Drink eight glasses of fresh, pure water every day.

'M DECLARING IT right now, so don't say I didn't warn you. This chapter's going to get juicy . . . a little risqué . . . a little, shall we say, *alternative*. A little *raw*. I'm going to talk to you about the joys, dare I call them the *glories*, of going naked, getting passionate, letting it all hang out. It's going to get downright X-rated . . . as in, X-tremely delicious.

But fear not! You needn't cover the children's eyes or close the book for fear of corrupting yourself. This chapter is also G-rated and pure as the driven snow (or as pure as the driven snow *used to be*). Because this chapter is about eating raw food.

MY RAW DEAL

I wasn't always such a big fan of raw food, but now I'm a true believer—not the extreme kind, but the Real Mom kind, who knows a good thing when she sees it. Here's how I learned the naked truth.

Several years ago, a dear friend of mine, Bonita, suggested that I attend a seminar led by a woman named Karyn Calabrese. Karyn is the owner of Karyn's Raw Café and Karyn's Inner Beauty Center in Chicago, and knowing just a little about the restaurant's reputation, I assumed the seminar would be about eating healthy food, cutting down on fat, eating more fruits and vegetables, taking supplements, yadda, yadda, yadda, all those things I already knew. I was already eating organic food, lots of fruits and vegetables, lean meats and salmon. What else was there? Still, I was looking for answers. Surely there was something else I could do to trim down that subcutaneous layer of fat I'd been carrying around since college. Like an old friend, it's been with me through thick and not-so-thin.

What I didn't expect was Karyn.

This woman was stunning. Light seemed to radiate from her, I swear. She had the most mesmerizing smile, the clearest, brightest eyes, the most beautiful strong body, the most gorgeous long hair. She had a calm energy that made everyone feel relaxed and alert. Most amazing of all, Karyn was old enough to be my *mother* . . . and yet she looked younger than most women my age. What was her secret? I had to know.

I listened attentively and couldn't believe what I was hearing. Karyn was excited and passionate about *food*, wonderful food—but not boring diet food. Not plain lean chicken with brown rice and steamed vegetables, hold the salt. She didn't suggest we skip dessert or exercise more or any of that. She had just one infatuation: *raw food.*

And not just any raw food. Not steak tartare or sashimi or raw eggs or even artisanal raw-milk cheeses. No, this gorgeous sixty-something woman was infatuated with raw living food: greens and crunchy, brightly colored vegetables, sweet jewel-colored fruits and their nectarlike juices. I confess, the way she talked about raw food got me very excited. If eating like this could make me look like *that*, well, then sign me up!

So I did sign up for Karyn's four-week green detox class. We met once a week for two hours, and I listened as Karyn dispelled myth after myth about eating raw food. She was intriguing and blunt, and most of all, she just had something I wanted—she *glowed*.

So, what was the plan? Each week built on the week before, making the program doable for busy moms. First, we were instructed to cut out all soda, white flour, and sugar from our diets while detoxing. Check, check, and check. What was next? Raw food—beautiful, green, fresh raw food, full of enzymes and phytochemicals and other seemingly magical properties that made Karyn practically sparkle like a member of the Cullen family out for a stroll in the sun (that's a *Twilight* reference, for all you Real Moms who aren't into the teen vampire craze).

But more was happening to me during that program. Karyn unlocked something inside of me, an awareness, an understanding, and a whole new respect for the living, breathing world. I also think the proof is in the pudding—or the raw chocolate mousse (find a yummy recipe for raw cacao mousse on page 97). Karyn has helped hundreds of people heal from debilitating disease just by showing them how to do a strict raw-food detox and diet. I've seen firsthand that raw food has real power.

Besides, you know those days when you just don't want to turn on the oven? Raw food is a get-out-of-cooking-free card. When I want to whip up something quick and easy without relying on processed foods, I fire up my Vitamix blender (it lives on my countertop within easy reach), throw in a few raw ingredients, and violà—instant food.

After my initial success with the raw-food detox, I was inspired and vowed to continue eating raw as best I could. However, I've been a lifelong meat eater, and eating raw plant foods definitely presented some challenges. If I was home, making my own meals, I was fine, but the minute I joined others for dinner out or somebody was having a barbecue, I was sunk. The rousing scent of burgers sizzling on the backyard grill called me back, like a siren song, to the world of cooked food. I know myself, and in general, my body reacts best with a little bit of animal food now and again, in the form of lean meat or salmon.

So today, I enjoy my cooked food but I also enjoy lots of fresh raw food every day, and I really enjoy making raw-food recipes. It's fun! It's cooking without cooking. But it takes some time too—you have to soak all your seeds and nuts, and you always have to plan ahead. And if your whole family isn't on board, you have to make two separate meals at dinnertime. What a pain in the turnip!

Real Moms don't always have the time to make multiple meals—even when it's extremely healthful. Like any eating style, it takes planning and preparation to eat only raw food, and let's face it, the kids' mac and cheese sure looks delicious at times, doesn't it? And while kids can and should eat a lot of raw food, known as a "high raw" diet, it does take careful planning to properly nourish their growing bodies on an all-raw diet. (A wonderful Web site about a family that is living 100 percent raw is www.rawfamily.com. They share their story and offer tips and resources on how you can make raw-food eating work within your lifestyle. I read their book, *Raw Family*, years ago and was impressed.) My kids love some of my raw creations, but at other times they just want a burger. And that's okay. You don't have to go 100 percent raw to experience the real health benefits, and stressing out about staying on the diet is only going to lessen the health benefits you can gain by eating raw in the first place. So take what you want from the raw diet, and enjoy!

After I began my raw-food odyssey, I used to feel so guilty when I'd steal a bite of my husband's juicy steak. Now I realize that if I really want a bite, I should take it. My body knows best, and when I listen to my body, I end up eating the right foods, across the board—the right foods for me. That usually means a more balanced approach. I think it's more realistic and workable in my world. Only *you* can know what works for your body. For some people, all raw all the time works great. For others, not so much. Every "body" reacts differently to different diets. I have incorporated lots of energy-rich, life-force-enhancing raw foods into my diet every day, and that has made all the difference. I feel great eating raw, so why not give it a try and trust how you look and feel?

Real Moms should know that raw is good, cooked is good, and, above all, good health, nutrition, and digestion should be a priority, no matter the cooked-or-not state of your food. So listen to your body, pay attention to your energy level, notice your tummy "aches" and fluctuating moods, and although you don't have to show them to anybody else, watch your stools: They should be even textured, not too runny and not too hard (they shouldn't resemble pebbles!), and if you are eating plenty of good, fresh raw fruits and veggies, they will probably move on out a couple of times a day. When everything looks and feels normal, you are probably eating what's right for you. When things get out of whack (diarrhea, constipation, strange colors), look first to your plate.

Indulge yourself by preparing a few raw-food recipes, and you too can come out of the closet with your love affair with food at its sexiest—*naked*. The more you eat, the better you'll feel. Your hips will trim down and you'll probably be most pleasantly stunned by the changes in your skin.

And don't forget that raw can't work its wonders unless you are also cutting way, way back on processed food. It's a small price to pay for silkier hair, stronger nails, a dewy complexion, and the energy of a *much* younger woman with a twinkle in her eye.

Tell your husband to consider himself warned. . . .

Chocolate in the Raw

MANY RAW FOODISTS love chocolate, but you won't find them noshing on a Hershey bar. They go for the real, the raw, the unprocessed cacao. This is the real thing, people. This is chocolate *naked*—what's sexier than that?

When I first encountered raw cacao, I tasted it in chocolaty raw brownies that my friend Bonita made for me. It wasn't as sweet as the chocolate I'd had before. Instead, it had more of the rich, bittersweet taste of a very dark chocolate, with a full-flavored, nutty texture. What was this food of the gods? I wondered.

Bonita told me that all forms of chocolate start here. It all begins with a pod that grows on a tree in the Amazon rain forest. Inside the pod is a bean. Peel the bean to reveal cacao nibs—Mother Nature's chocolate chips! These nibs can be ground up to make raw cacao powder, which is similar to cocoa powder, but which is not roasted (hence the "raw" part). The higher the cacao content in your favorite chocolate bar, the more intense the chocolate flavor, the more

(continued)

YOUR RAW-FOOD TOOL KIT

There exists a world out there—a whole new, wondrous world of raw-food recipes. With cookbooks and online resources galore (just type "raw-food recipes" in your search engine), you can immerse yourself in a whole new raw dimension of culinary exploration.

However, anybody embarking on such a fantastic voyage needs to be well equipped. Raw-food "cooking" requires a few basic tools and ingredients that you will see referred to over and over again. Just consider me your raw-food Sherpa—here's your list of supplies:

TOOLS

* **VITAMIX (OR OTHER HEAVY-DUTY BLENDER):** Blenders are indispensable for transforming fruit into smoothies and making pureed soup, but of all the blenders out there in all the world, I recommend the Vitamix. It's so much more than just a blender. It's powerful, easy to use, and versatile. I can whip up a smoothie, pour it in a glass, then add water to the Vitamix pitcher and run it on low, and it cleans itself (oh, if only that worked for *all* my appliances!). Then I can add the ingredients for a soup and run it on high and it blends everything together, and even actually heats up the food because of the incredibly high blending speed. It can even grind up grains and nuts so you can make your own flour and nut meal.

The only issue some people have with the Vitamix is

cost. They can be pretty pricey—some models are over $500. However, unlike cheaper blenders that burn out in a few years, this is a blender to last a lifetime. (And if you're eating a lot of raw food, that's going to be a very, very long time!) I was able to get mine at a discounted price through a special on their Web site: www.Vitamix.com.

✳ **FOOD DEHYDRATOR:** My oven has a "dehydrate" mode. It's great—I make dehydrated fruit, flax crackers, and raw pizza crust. You can even make your own jerky. Or try yummy, crispy kale chips—delish! (Find the recipe on page 226.) If your oven isn't similarly equipped, you can purchase a dehydrator as a small appliance.

Dehydrating food enhances the flavor and makes it more vivid—and preserves it without the chemical preservatives and high salt content that are in so much processed food. When I'm dehydrating food (fruit, vegetables, leafy greens), I make sure to cut it down to quarter-inch-thick bite-size pieces so it dehydrates all the way through in the time required. This will keep it from getting gummy. Dehydrated food should be crisp and crunchy. I store the dehydrated food in airtight containers it has completely cooled, so that any residual moisture from the cooling process doesn't get trapped inside the container.

A great place to get one is www.fooddehydrators.com. They are as little as $29.99, although you can pay hundreds of dollars for a really fancy one, if you are so inclined. If you think you're going to prepare and eat dehydrated foods on a regular basis, it's definitely worth purchasing one. Or get one and share it with a friend.

✳ **SPIRALIZER OR MANDOLINE:** Many raw-food recipes require that veggies or fruits be thinly sliced, and while you can do that by hand with a good chef's knife, it's a heck of a lot easier if you have a handy gadget like a spiralizer or a mandoline. Using various attachments, a mandoline can slice a zucchini, a tomato, or an apple in seconds, giving you beautiful, uniform slices. A spiralizer slices vegetables into long thin strips—veggie noodles! I highly recommend these tools as time-savers, and just for aesthetic reasons, to make your raw food more beautiful and appealing. They are particularly handy for one of my favorite recipes, Raw Lasagna (see page 92).

* **DEDICATED SPICE GRINDER:** I dedicate one of my coffee grinders to cooking. I use it to grind flaxseeds, nuts, and spices like cumin seeds, for the freshest possible taste (whether for raw recipes or not). Since I use flaxseeds in my smoothie every day, I usually grind enough to last me for a few days. Always keep ground flaxseeds in a covered glass container in the refrigerator so they stay fresh.

* **SOAKING JAR:** Most raw foodists recommend soaking nuts, seeds, and even some grains and legumes before eating. Soaking activates the dormant enzymes in these foods by initiating the sprouting process. A large mason jar or something similar with a lid should do the trick.

INGREDIENTS

Raw-food recipes are full of diversity, but there are a few ingredients you see time and time again. Keeping them around means you'll always be ready to whip up something raw and wonderful. Make sure to have:

* Fresh leafy greens and seasonal raw vegetables
* Seasonal fruit
* Avocados
* Raw cacao powder and nibs
* A variety of raw nuts and seeds
* Raw almonds, for making almond milk
* A variety of unsulfured dried raw fruit, especially pitted dates, but also figs, raisins, apricots, and other fruits that don't contain added sugar. (Unsulfured means sulfur was not used as a preservative in processing, i.e., the fruit doesn't contain this additive. I wish more dried fruits were sugar-free—read the label! Your natural food store will be more likely to carry the truly natural stuff.)

* Raw agave nectar
* Raw shredded coconut

Raw = Green

EVERY TIME YOU eat a fresh, living, raw food, you are doing something to help protect the planet. Raw food does not require long cooking or prep times (except when you dehydrate, but dehydrating is on low, low temps—90 to 105 degrees), so the energy used to prepare it is virtually nil. If you buy local produce, the energy to transport it is much lower than it would be if you were buying exotic fruits and vegetables shipped from far away.

Eating raw food locally in season is greener still, because you are not just getting food at its fresh best, but supporting a process of agriculture that has minimal impact. When you take yet another step and buy organic, you are voting with your dollars to keep pesticides and other agriculture chemicals *out of the food chain.*

So even if you don't eat all raw, every raw piece of fruit or vegetable you consume is a little hug for Mother Earth.

DO FIVE THINGS

Are you inspired? Are you ready to get naked? Are you ready to launch week five on the Real Moms Love to Eat plan? Great! This week, your tasks will largely consist of adding *something* (anything!) raw to every meal of every day. I include some mind-blowing yummy recipes from two dear friends: personal fitness trainer, raw-food chef, and anti-aging coach Bonita Kindle (www.rawfoodsandfitness.com) and raw-food chef extraordinaire Susie Sondag (www.HipGoddess. com). Specifically, here's what I want you to do this week:

1. ADD SOMETHING RAW TO EVERY BREAKFAST.

The easiest way to add something raw to breakfast is to eat fresh raw fruit. Simple! Just slice an orange or a grapefruit, nibble on some berries, or bite into an apple. Fruit is the ultimate fast food. But you can be more creative too. I already gave you my favorite smoothie recipe in chapter one, but smoothies are ultimately versatile. Breakfast is a great time to experiment with new ingredients and flavors.

One of my raw-food guru Karyn's favorite recipes is her green smoothie. She makes and sells a powdered green mix that I always use called the Green Meal (you can find it on her Web site at www.karynraw.com/products). The smoothie is a blast of nutrients. Here's how she makes it:

KARYN'S GREEN SMOOTHIE

1 scoop Green Meal
½ cup pure organic apple juice
½ cup coconut water
1 frozen banana
1 tablespoon lecithin granules
1 heaping tablespoon of ground flaxseeds

1. Sometimes I'll also add a tablespoon each of flax oil and a vanilla protein powder

2. Blend everything together in your Vitamix or blender and sip to your heart's content.

2. ADD SOMETHING RAW TO EVERY LUNCH.

Lunch is easy too. All you need is a big fresh salad full of leafy greens and raw vegetables, extra virgin olive oil, and a squeeze of citrus juice. But that's not your only option. I have three sons and a hungry husband to feed, and on most days, a plain old salad isn't going to cut it. I'm often driving all over the city to drop off my sons at all their athletic activities, and then I've also got to get some food in them without resorting to the fast-food drive-through.

Bonita found the perfect option for me, and I make it regularly: raw nut pâté. This is so easy to make that you may want to whip up a batch a couple of times a week. Store it in a glass container and enjoy it anytime, lickety-split. Lunchtime: solved!

Here's how to make it:

RAW NUT PÂTÉ

1 cup tree nuts (almonds, walnuts, cashews, or a mixture), soaked
    overnight in purified water in a bowl or jar with a lid, then
    drained
1 roma tomato, sliced
½ onion, peeled
Sea salt, to taste

Put all the ingredients in your Vitamix or food processor and blend until creamy. If the paste seems too thick, add a little bit of water, a tablespoon at a time, to get the consistency you want. Scoop it onto a plate covered in Bibb or romaine lettuce leaves and surround it with carrot sticks, green pepper strips, celery stalks, zucchini spears, cucumber slices, or other favorite raw veggies. You can also top the pâté with a little bit of grated carrot, chopped fresh parsley or cilantro, or a dash of paprika, for color and style.

3. ADD SOMETHING RAW TO EVERY DINNER.

Adding something raw to dinner is a no-brainer if you whip up a big salad for every meal, and getting into the salad habit really is one of the best things you can do for your diet. But why stop there? There are hundreds of fun raw foods you can try for dinner, literally from soup to nuts. One of my favorite recipes, actually one of my all-time favorite dinners, is Bonita's raw lasagna, which I featured recently on my Web site (www.realmomslovetoeat.com). It's not what it sounds like! You have to think outside the . . . lasagna pan. This recipe is so delicious, I get tongue-tied just thinking about it.

Bonita warned me that I would need only about a three-inch square, because the flavors and living enzymes in this dish are so intense. I didn't heed her warning, of course—I was starving!—and I doubled my serving. Halfway through, I had to agree with her that the intense flavors were something I'd never experienced before. The party going on in my mouth was so decadently sensual and pure, such a sinfully innocent orgy of taste, that I barely knew which way was up! Even though I didn't think the recipe made that much, I was able to eat the leftovers for three days.

Here's how to make it:

🍳 SEXY RAW LASAGNA

■ SERVES 6 TO 8.

FOR THE CASHEW CHEESE:
1 cup raw cashews, soaked in purified water in a covered glass
    jar or bowl for at least 4 hours or overnight, drained
Juice squeezed from 1 fresh lemon
¾ teaspoon sea salt

FOR THE TOMATO SAUCE:
1 to 2 cloves garlic (depending on how much you love garlic)
2 to 4 leaves of fresh basil
1 small jar of sun-dried tomatoes in olive oil (or use bagged sun-
    dried tomatoes and let them soak for about 15 minutes in 1
    tablespoon olive oil)
1 roma tomato, or ½ regular tomato

FOR ASSEMBLING THE LASAGNA:
3 medium zucchini
3 cups fresh spinach, coarsely chopped
1 tablespoon chopped fresh (or 1 teaspoon dried) oregano

1. Make the cashew "cheese": Put the cashews, lemon juice, and salt in a food processor and process until smooth. Add up to 1 tablespoon water if it's too thick. Set aside.

2. Make the sauce: In the bowl of a food processor, add the garlic. Process until chopped, just a few pulses. Add the basil leaves and process until chopped, just a few pulses. Add the sun-dried tomato and fresh tomato. Process until smooth.

3. Assemble the lasagna: Slice the zucchini lengthwise to make long thin "noodle" slices. (The mandoline makes quick work of this task.) In the bottom of a glass baking pan that is approximately 8" x 8" put ⅓ of the zucchini slices. Spread ⅓ of the cashew "cheese" over the zucchini. Sprinkle ⅓ of the chopped spinach over the "cheese." Pour ⅓ of the sauce over the spinach. Repeat two more times to use all the ingredients. Sprinkle oregano on top.

4. To serve, cut the lasagna into *small* squares. Add a big fresh salad and raw flax crackers (see recipe on page 96), or a good loaf of fresh whole-grain bread, if you want your dinner to be (literally) half-baked. Store in the refrigerator for up to three or four days.

━━━━━

4. KEEP THREE DIFFERENT RAW SNACKS YOU REALLY LIKE IN YOUR KITCHEN AT ALL TIMES.

Snacks are probably the easiest way to eat raw—just grab a piece of fruit or a handful of precut veggies. But the options go beyond the apple-or-baby-carrots conundrum. Other yummy raw snacks to keep in stock and easy to find:

* **RAW NUTS:** I keep bowls accessible, filled with raw almonds, walnuts, and cashews. With protein and the good kind of fat, nuts keep you satisfied for a long time. You might also want to keep a small snack bag of nuts in your purse at all times, when you find yourself starving and stuck in traffic or nowhere near any other healthy food.
* **FINGER FRUIT:** This is what I call fruit you can grab with your fingers and eat like candy—blueberries, raspberries, grapes. Or make finger fruit by slicing melons, apples, or banana wheels, or sectioning oranges. If it's ready to eat, you and your kids will be more likely to grab it.

* **FRUIT WITH BUILT-IN HANDLES:** An apple, a banana, a bunch of grapes on the stem are all easy to take with you, and fill you up.

* **VEGGIES THAT CAN TRAVEL WITHOUT GETTING BRUISED:** Like pea pods, edamame, and, of course, those old standbys, baby carrots and celery stalks. Or splurge on store-bought precut veggies, if you just can't find the time (or energy) to rinse and chop the broccoli, cauliflower, green peppers, and carrots. I also like that premade broccoli-carrot slaw in bags. Just toss with a bit of balsamic vinaigrette or your favorite salad dressing, pop it in a travel container, and you've got a snack all ready to go.

* **RAW ENERGY BARS:** I love LÄRABAR brand, made with dried fruit and nuts in the most delectable flavors: cherry pie, cinnamon roll, peanut butter and jelly, and many more. My go-to snack bar.

* **LEFTOVER NUT PÂTÉ:** (Recipe on page 91.) In mini containers with sliced veggies.

* **PITTED DATES:** With a raw almond or pecan shoved inside— you'll almost think you're eating pecan pie, no kidding!

* **PREMADE TRAIL MIX STORED IN MINI CONTAINERS:** My favorite combination is walnuts, cashews, raisins, dried cranberries, cacao nibs, and just a dash of sea salt. Try your own combinations using your favorite nuts, seeds, dried fruit, raw cracker bits, etc. Trail mix is another great purse food.

* **RAW POPSICLES:** Make sun tea in a glass pitcher using green and/or hibiscus tea (my favorites), then add the juice of a whole lemon. Stir in a little bit of agave nectar or honey and pour into ice cube trays or ice-pop molds to make homemade raw ice pops.

* **MELON:** In the summer, blend an entire melon (not the rind, of course) in your Vitamix or blender until it's pure juice. Store in a glass pitcher for a cleansing and refreshing snack in a glass.

* **RAW FLAXSEED CRACKERS:** These are so easy to make if you have a dehydrator—they are chewy and tasty. Here are two versions:

SWEET CINNAMON FLAX CRACKERS

■ MAKES APPROXIMATELY 2 DOZEN.

½ cup water
2 cups flaxseeds soaked 12 hours in 3½ cups water (do not rinse
or drain)
1 tablespoon ground cinnamon
1 tablespoon agave nectar

1. Transfer the soaked flaxseeds to a large bowl, add the agave nectar and cinnamon, and stir well to combine.

2. Spread the 2½ cups of flaxseed "batter" about ⅛-inch thick on a Silpat cookie sheet liner; then place liner onto dehydrator pans. It's much easier to spread the batter on the liners before you place them on the "wavy" dehydrator trays—trust me!

3. Score the crackers into squares and dehydrate at 115 degrees for 12 hours.

4. Flip the crackers onto just the dehydrator sheet and continue to dehydrate another 12 hours or until completely dry.

5. Allow crackers to cool and store in covered glass bowls. Crackers will keep all week long at room temperature.

SAVORY PIZZA FLAX CRACKERS

■ **MAKES 2 DOZEN.**

¾ cup sun-dried tomatoes (preferably packed in oil)
½ cup water
1½ cup chopped red bell pepper
¼ cup chopped onion
2 cloves of garlic, crushed
1 teaspoon lemon juice
1¼ teaspoon sea salt
1 teaspoon Italian seasoning
¼ cup minced fresh basil
2 cups flaxseeds soaked 12 hours in 3½ cups water (do not rinse
     or drain)

1. In the jar of your blender or food processor, combine the sun-dried tomatoes and water and blend to form a paste. Add red bell pepper, onion, garlic, lemon juice, and salt. Blend or process, adding additional water to thin if necessary; add fresh herbs and pulse to mix.

2. Transfer the vegetable mixture to a large bowl, add the soaked flaxseeds, and stir well to combine.

3. Spread the 2½ cups of flaxseed "batter" about ⅛-inch thick on a Silpat cookie sheet liner, then place liner onto dehydrator pans.

4. Score the crackers into squares, then dehydrate at 115 degrees for 12 hours.

5. Flip the crackers onto the dehydrator sheet and continue to dehydrate another 12 hours or until completely dry. Allow crackers to cool and store in covered glass bowls—crackers will keep all week long at room temperature.

AND WHAT ABOUT DESSERT?

So many luscious raw desserts, so little time . . . Here are two of my favorites.

TASTY LEMON-CASHEW FREEZER COOKIES

Combine 2 cups soaked cashews, ¼ cup agave nectar, 3 tablespoons freshly squeezed lemon juice, 2½ tablespoons freshly grated and finely chopped lemon zest, 1 teaspoon vanilla extract, and ¼ teaspoon sea salt in the blender or food processor until it forms a dough. Form it into a roll with your hands and slice. Keep these cookies in the freezer for those sweet-tooth moments.

SLINKY, SULTRY RAW CHOCOLATE MOUSSE

Combine 3 ripe organic bananas, 4 to 5 tablespoons of raw cacao powder, 1 small avocado, 1 teaspoon coconut water, ¼ teaspoon vanilla extract, 3 to 4 drops liquid stevia (optional, if the bananas aren't sweet enough for you). Blend everything in the Vitamix or food processor until smooth. Serve in fancy glasses with a few cacao nibs sprinkled on top for garnish.

5. DRINK EIGHT GLASSES OF FRESH, PURE WATER EVERY DAY.

You are now at your target water consumption to keep yourself well hydrated, your skin dewy, and your eyes bright. Although many raw foods contain a lot of water, and you might not always want eight full glasses every day when you are eating lots of fruits and vegetables, eight glasses is a great target. So keep yourself well juiced up with good old H_2O!

Phew! Was that chapter as good for you as it was for me? Naked raw food really will make you feel sexier, better nourished, and all around *sweeter*; plus it means cooking *less*. Even after the week is over, continue to eat raw whenever you can. Your inner nature girl will thank you. You'll see a difference in your weight, skin, hair, energy level, and attitude. And you'll positively glow with radiance. What's not to love about that?

CHAPTER
SIX

WEEK SIX:

Find Your Sweet Spot

THIS WEEK, DO FIVE THINGS:

1. Try a new dessert made of fruit.
2. Try a new chocolate recipe with a natural sweetener.
3. Reserve sweet foods for only one time per day. Make it special!
4. Try juicing. I'll get you started.
5. Keep drinking your eight glasses of fresh, pure water every day.

YOU KNOW THAT feeling you get when you realize you're being seduced . . . and it's working? You get those butterflies in your chest, that little smile you can't quite suppress. You have trouble concentrating as you picture the object of your desire, as the longing in the pit of your stomach grows. You think about the pleasure and you get tingles. You feel worshiped; you feel like you have superpowers; you feel like the most decadently indulged woman on the planet.

This is how I feel about cupcakes.

Lest you mistake my reverie for guilt, let me assure you that I hereby refuse to feel guilty about pleasure. Getting sick from eating three cupcakes is not pleasurable. Really making love to one perfect cupcake *is*. Because you know what?

Eating a cupcake is not a crime!

Neither is eating a cookie or a brownie or a piece of birthday or wedding cake. Neither is savoring a piece of candy or indulging in a warm piece of pie *with ice cream*!

Deprivation isn't a crime either, *but it should be.*

It's too bad that this is even an issue, but for a lot of Real Moms, it is. We've been brought up from a young age to think that eating sweets is somehow a bad thing. We feel guilty. We think we are being bad. *There is nothing bad about sweets.* What's bad is overindulging, crossing over to the dark side by making yourself miserable and guilty because you ate more than your body really wanted.

I believe the reason some women overdo it when it comes to sweets is simply that we can't get over the notion that we *aren't allowed to have them*, and some part of us rebels. If all the restrictions disappeared, if you really, truly believed from the bottom of your heart and the base of your brain that you could eat any pleasurable food you wanted to eat without any guilt or remorse, not even a twinge, would you really eat the entire plate of cookies? Would you really go through the whole party-size bag of M&M's? Or would you have no problem stopping at one or two cookies, or a small handful of candy-coated chocolates? (Have you tried the new coconut M&M's? Just when you thought M&Ms were perfect? But I digress. . . .)

So this is the root of the problem: You think it's bad, so you tell yourself no, and then, like a rebellious toddler, the first thing you want to do is the thing that you aren't supposed to do. So you eat too much, in rebellion, in frustration. And then you feel guilty, horrible, sick. You vow never to eat sugar again. *No more sugar for you!* And then the cycle starts all over again.

Girlfriends, it's time to make a jailbreak. Whether your weakness is gummi bears, cheesecake, chocolate croissants, apple fritters, jelly beans, Dove bars, or your special holiday fudge (have you ever made it with chopped almonds and dried cherries and a dash of amaretto? Mind-blowing! But I digress again . . .), it's time to stand up with me, hold up your right hand, and repeat:

I like sweets and I'm not afraid to eat them!
I like sweets and it's perfectly normal to want them!
I like sweets and I'm going to have them whenever
  I really want them!

What's with the chirping crickets in the background? Why isn't anybody joining in?

Oh, I see. You're scared. If you say those words, you think you'll go out of control. You'll lose it. You'll become a candy junkie. You'll never eat another vegetable. You'll gain fifty pounds in a week. I can almost hear the panicky fantasies going on in your head.

Look, Real Moms: There is one reason you go overboard on the Raisinets and the Junior Mints and the Toll House cookies. No, it's not because they contain carbs. It's not because sugar is poison. It's not because you're going to start mainlining frosting. It's because you are telling yourself that you really can't have sweets, and you might never get any again. In a panic, fearing deprivation, you go overboard the other way and load up, just in case it's the last chance you're ever going to get to enjoy a Snickers bar.

When you let go, really let go of this deprivation mentality, sweets lose their power over you. You can still love them, adore them, want to spend the weekend at their place with the phone off the hook, but they won't control you anymore.

There is a big difference between love and obsession. One is fun. The other isn't.

So let's keep it fun, Real Moms. Let's loosen up the reins and chill out and recognize that sugar can be a wonderfully sweet part of your life without being the only part. It's sugar; it's not air. It's for pleasure, not survival. I'm going to show you how to enjoy it without letting it hurt you anymore.

GOD'S CANDY

Candy is dandy and liquor may be quicker, as they say, but of all the sweet sensations on the planet, Real Moms must know the truth: All the man-made sweets ever made are pale imitations of the original candy, God's candy.

I'm talking about fruit.

Fruit is the whole package. It is the original sugar. It is smart and nutritious, wholesome and mighty fine-looking, at that. Fruit has everything you ever wished you could bring home to your parents to impress them. It's the Harvard grad with the double major in finance and poetry, who's fluent in six languages and loves kids and also just finished med school but wants to support your career. Fruit is practically perfect.

Growing up, I would watch my mom eat fruit nonstop. She just loved it, especially with a light sprinkle of sugar on top—and why the heck not? Now her yard is full of fruit trees, but she also buys fruit in season. Her house is always full of the juiciest, most delectable fruit on the planet.

I remember waking up in the morning and finding the remains of half a watermelon, complete with little black seeds and drying pink liquid on the plate. Mom and Dad had obviously been enjoying a late-night snack. Now I know that watermelon has a diuretic effect, which comes in handy when you want something sweet and you *also* want to deflate your belly for a day at the beach. Watermelon is cleansing, nourishing, and full of lycopene, a potent antioxidant.

My mom also loved to make bowls of blueberries and cut strawberries. Just recently I was at her house. She had piles of berries on the counter, just for me. She likes to slice up the strawberries in little pieces and sprinkle them with sugar. As the sugar coaxes the juice out of the berries, they begin to swim in a red-pink syrup—perfect for topping a slice of angel food cake.

Feeling Blue?

RECENTLY, I DID a news segment for ABC-7 in Chicago about food for beautiful skin. One of my most enthusiastic recommendations was blueberries, because they are such a perfect antiaging food. I've been eating them for years, but only recently did I decide to do a bit of research on what makes these babies so superior. Sure

(continued)

enough, they are loaded with antioxidants like anthocyanin, vitamin A, B-complex vitamins, and vitamins C and E, as well as copper, zinc, selenium, and iron. They may help boost the immune system, oxygenate the blood, manage cholesterol, improve vision, and burn belly fat. What an awesome berry! No box of candy can claim stats like that.

So when I think of dessert, I always try to include blueberries, whenever they are in season, whether it's a fresh bowl of raw berries with whipped cream or a yummy, healthful Peach-blueberry Crumble. (Find the recipe on page 106.)

The reason fruit is such a superior form of sugar is that it has luscious sweetness but also fiber, vitamins, and minerals, so it's a more natural way to get your sweet fix, a way your body understands and can digest more easily and smoothly.

Fruit is also versatile. You can eat it raw or cook it and eat it warm; you can bake it into a hot pie or cobbler or crisp or muffin, or blend it into an ice-cold smoothie or milk shake.

Fruit is never more sensual than when it is at its seasonal peak— the first blushing strawberries in the spring, the juicy midsummer nectarine season, the first crisp fall apples ready to be plucked, or the long-awaited shipment of grapefruit and oranges in the winter.

When you want something sweet, always remember fruit first. You may not decide to go with it, but think about how you can buy a candy bar any old time of year, but this July, the plums are absolutely perfect, and they won't last for long.

RECLAIMING WHAT'S SPECIAL

Finally, I want to talk about something that I believe is very important, but which our society seems to have forgotten: the value of keeping something special. Remember when you were a kid, and every once in a while, like on Halloween or a winter holiday, you got some candy? Or you saved your allowance so you could go buy some on your own, and it tasted so perfectly sweet that it practically defines your memories of childhood?

What happened to those days?

Today kids get candy all the time. They get it at home, at friends' houses, even in school! I've heard of kids getting rewarded for turning in their homework with candy bars from the teacher. What the heck?

Where once kids marveled at the special occasions that warranted sweets, today sweets seem to be expected. Whoever said we were entitled to that kind of pleasure twenty-four/seven? When you eat sugar all day, every day, it isn't special anymore. It's just a habit.

You know that feeling when you wake up in the morning so excited because you know you are going to do something really rare and wonderful that day? Maybe it's date night with your husband and you're going out to dinner and a movie you've been dying to see. Maybe it's girls' night out. Maybe you're going on a trip, or it's a special holiday. Looking forward to something rare and wonderful puts me in a good mood all day long (although my friends will probably tell you I'm always like that anyway—they call me "think-positive girl"). Knowing I'm going to be wined and dined or have much-needed friend time or get to go somewhere new makes me feel so great.

Sweets should be like that.

It could be the worst rainy, cold day where everything goes wrong and you're really feeling the stress, the washing machine is on the blink, your dog is throwing up on the carpet, and you can feel a sore throat coming on. But what if you also knew that precisely at seven p.m., you had an unbreakable date, just you, a glass of wine, a perfect brownie (with frosting!), and a bubble bath? Wouldn't that make your day feel a little bit sweeter?

Eating sweets all day will make you feel more stressed out because your blood sugar will head off on a roller-coaster ride and you'll be Mrs. Mood Swings. Mainlining sweets that way is literally spoiling yourself, but eating sweets every once in a while, even just one time in a day, can fill you with expectation and appreciation for the good things in life—the things you really let yourself savor. That's celebrating yourself, and that's exactly what Real Moms should do.

Wholesome Sweets

SOMETIMES SWEETS ARE purely an indulgence, a way to enjoy yourself, a *pleasure*. But that doesn't mean they can't also be nutritious. There are so many ways to up the nutrient profile of sweets, so that every calorie counts. Why throw away a two-hundred-calorie snack on candy when you could have all the pleasure plus fiber, vitamins, and minerals? What if you could cut that snack to a hundred calories without tasting the difference? Real Moms *require* good fuel to run on, so they don't run out before the kids do.

There are many ways to do this. You just have to think before you nosh. For example, baking with whole-grain pastry flour, natural sweeteners, and healthful additions like oatmeal, wheat germ, nuts, and dried fruit can turn dessert into something truly nourishing. Many of the dessert recipes in this book will show you how to transform your favorite sweets from nutritionally so-so to nutritionally spectacular, so you can have your proverbial cake and benefit from it too.

DO FIVE THINGS

Real Moms, it's time to revamp your relationship with the sweet stuff. So many diets tell you to get all sweets out of your house, but when we forbid ourselves, not to mention our kids, to do something, the power of that thing grows. We all want what we can't have. So in my house I make sure we all eat a healthy balance of protein, complex carbohydrates, fruits and vegetables, and healthy fats. Then, when the topic of dessert or sweet snacks comes up, I can usually say, "Yes!" When sweets aren't omnipresent but aren't off-limits either, they can be a regular, delicious part of an overall healthy diet, especially when you juice them up to be extra nutritious.

This week, do these five things, and feel yourself getting steadier, calmer, and more deeply appreciative of everything sweet in your life.

1. TRY A NEW DESSERT MADE OF FRUIT.

This week, I want you to give fruit some love. Restore it to its rightful place as a dessert. *Honor it* by incorporating it into one delicious dessert this week.

There are so many options. Every year I look forward to peach season, because one of my very favorite sweet things is Real Mom Peach-blueberry Crumble, a dessert I adapted from a recipe called Navajo Peach Crumble from *Moosewood Restaurant Book of Desserts*, by Mollie Katzen. When the first bags of fresh, ripe peaches become available at my farmers' market, I get so excited, because it means I get to make my first crumble of the season. Which leads to another. And another. Until the peaches are gone for another year (sniff).

This recipe is easy and foolproof. The result is a soul-satisfying dessert that works as well for an informal brunch in your pajamas as it does for a fancy dinner party. (And I'm always up for one of those—your place? What time shall I arrive? I'll bring the crumble!)

Here's what you do:

REAL MOM PEACH-BLUEBERRY CRUMBLE

■ SERVES 4.

½ cup whole-wheat pastry flour
½ cup whole-grain cornmeal
⅔ cup raw sugar or maple sugar, divided in half
⅛ teaspoon sea salt
⅓ cup butter, cut into little chunks
2 cups peeled, sliced peaches (or nectarines, apples, pears, or
     any kind of berry)
1 cup blueberries
1 teaspoon cinnamon
Dash of nutmeg
Juice of one lemon, freshly squeezed

1. Preheat the oven to 375 degrees. In a small bowl, combine the flour, cornmeal, ⅓ cup of the sugar, the salt, and butter. Mash it up with a fork or pastry blender until it is in coarse crumbs, or give it a few pulses in your food processor.

2. In a glass pie pan, combine the fruit, the remaining sugar, lemon juice, cinnamon, and nutmeg. Stir everything together. Sprinkle the topping evenly over it.

3. Bake until the fruit is bubbling and the topping is golden brown, about 30 minutes.

4. Serve warm, with or without ice cream.

WATERMELON SMOOTHIE

For those days when you want something fruity and sweet but you don't have time to bake a dessert (like . . . *every day*?), try a watermelon smoothie. This is probably the simplest smoothie ever. Put a few big hunks of watermelon meat, scooped from the rind, into the blender. Blend. Add a few more hunks. Blend again. Drink.

This smoothie is the very essence of watermelon, an awesome source of vitamins A and C and other antioxidants that travel through the body fast, neutralizing free radicals. And remember what I said about the debloating power of everybody's favorite melon?

2. TRY A NEW CHOCOLATE RECIPE WITH NATURAL SWEETENER.

Can we give chocolate a loving moment of silence, please?

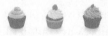

Okay, that was good. Because sometimes I just have to thank chocolate for existing. You can't possibly have read this far into the book without having a pretty good idea of how chocolate and I feel about each other. It's one of those affairs that lasts a lifetime.

I still love custard pie and vanilla ice cream; don't get me wrong. I'm not hating on those delicious and creamy desserts, especially when they are topped with bright, fresh berries. However, since my hubby introduced me to dark chocolate, my love for it has grown exponentially. I'm like Anakin Skywalker, getting ever closer to the dark side of the Force—but in a *good* way! Because chocolate isn't just good. It's good for you, and the darker, the better. I'm talking Darth Vader dark. (Hey, that would be a great name for a new chocolate bar!)

I remember when I first got married and never gave a thought to gaining weight. My husband and I would eat a full three-course dinner and then share the colossal Black-Out Cake at the Cheesecake Factory. And we could still finish our extra-tall sweetened iced teas! We worked out regularly at Chicago's trendy East Bank Club two hours a day. (Yes, you are correct—we didn't yet have any kids. And I was ripped; I kid you not. I'm talking six-pack abs.) We also went running together along the city's lakefront on weekends, and we played in a beach volleyball league every Wednesday night, where I could flex my mean underhand serve.

But as anyone who was once newly married and is now comfortably married with a child or two under her belt (and carrying a little extra baggage under that belt) can guess, birth by exhilarating birth, my metabolism slowed down and the joys of motherhood took the place of the joys of beach volleyball and daily gym time.

I still trained for marathons during this time, and ran four of them, but I typically trained with a double stroller during the week to get my miles in. My husband would watch our sons on the weekends while I did the long runs. But even then I began to realize I could no longer eat with the same kind of reckless abandon that had characterized those over-the-top Cheesecake Factory meals.

My body just didn't want to let go of the body fat around my hips and thighs, marathon or no marathon. Like a Ping-Pong ball across a table, I bounced up and down, breaking up and getting back together with the same twenty pounds for years. Talk about a dysfunctional relationship. Why couldn't I move on? I had to make a decision, or so I thought: slim thighs or colossal chocolate cake. Which did I want more? Who would have to go?

Then, one year after the birth of my third son, I had my introduction to raw food (see chapter five) and incorporating whole foods into my diet (see chapter eight), and that changed everything. Suddenly, after years of pain from irritable bowel syndrome, my digestive system calmed down and began to run more smoothly. My skin cleared up and I had a ton of energy. And I found that I didn't crave chocolate with the same intensity as I had before. I began to see chocolate as a special friend I could meet up with now and again for some fun, rather than as something I had to sneak around to see, then feel guilty about. When I enjoyed chocolate raw, it agreed with me more—and was better for me too.

I'm not saying you can't have chocolate cake. You *can* have chocolate cake, when you really want it, when you really think it will be worth it, when you know it will make you feel good instead of bad, and when you can trust yourself to know when enough is enough.

To practice indulging in chocolate smartly (and more often!), this week I want you to make one chocolate dessert with natural sweetener, like this Deep Dark Delicious Chocolate Sauce. Instead of promising you the moon and then hurting your belly all night (I'm talking to you, Black-Out Cake!), this will actually make you feel great. And it couldn't be easier.

This chocolate spoonful of love was introduced to me by my dear "sweet" friend Susie, who, like my friends Bonita and Karyn, is a great resource for me when it comes to raw-food eating and recipes!

DEEP DARK DELICIOUS CHOCOLATE SAUCE

■ **SERVES 1; CAN EASILY BE DOUBLED OR TRIPLED FOR MORE SERVINGS.**

2 tablespoons raw agave syrup
½ teaspoon coconut oil
2 tablespoons raw cacao powder

Mix the agave syrup and oil together with a spoon or whisk. Slowly whisk the raw cacao powder into the syrup mixture until well blended. Do not use a food processor or Vitamix for this recipe—it must be done by hand. Drizzle over . . . anything! (Well, maybe not broccoli.)

Is that too simple? Or not enough? You want to make *more* chocolate desserts? I can hardly blame you. I do too—so how about a most delicious sugar-free chocolate-chip banana bread? This recipe is great for when you've got overripe bananas. They are so fruity-sweet that you don't even need sugar. Make this recipe and you've knocked out your fruit dessert *and* your natural chocolate dessert requirements for the week.

Maybe you'd better make a couple of batches . . . because this is really good for breakfast too.

My friend Jane whips up this recipe of hers whenever she has a hankering for something sweet, but still wants to eat something healthy.

FRUIT-SWEET CHOCOLATE-CHIP BANANA BREAD

■ **MAKES ONE LOAF.**

3 or 4 overripe bananas
1 tablespoon fresh lemon juice
½ cup melted butter or canola oil
¾ cup real maple syrup
1½ cups whole-wheat pastry flour
½ cup wheat germ
½ teaspoon salt
½ teaspoon baking soda
½ teaspoon baking powder
½ cup dark chocolate chips or cacao nibs

1. Preheat the oven to 375 degrees. In a large bowl, mash the ripe bananas with a fork. Add the lemon juice, butter or oil, and maple syrup. Mix until thoroughly combined.

2. In another large bowl, combine the flour, wheat germ, salt, baking soda, baking powder, and chocolate chips or nibs. Add the wet ingredients and stir just until combined.

3. Pour the batter into a lightly oiled loaf pan and bake for 40 to 50 minutes, or until a toothpick inserted into the center of the loaf comes out clean or with just a few moist crumbs. Cool on a wire rack for at least one hour (if you can stand it). Slice and serve, or wrap up and store in the freezer or refrigerator.

3. RESERVE SWEET FOODS FOR ONLY ONE TIME PER DAY. MAKE IT SPECIAL!

Sweets are special. It's a simple concept, holistic and pure. When you elevate sweets to that special, honored position in your day, they become what they are meant to be—lovely little indulgences to keep you going. So this week, I want you to enjoy something sweet every day . . . but *only once*. Fruit doesn't count. You can eat fruit for every meal, as far as I'm concerned. I'm talking about desserts with sugar—cookies, brownies, cake, candy, chocolate, or sugary soda. Have a perfect, special time you set aside just for yourself to savor and enjoy something sweet, whether it's midmorning with your coffee, midafternoon when you can't wait until dinner, or in the evening, to help you relax and wind down after a long day.

Eating something sweet just once a day will condition you to appreciate the little pleasures in life. Soon you may find you get less annoyed when your husband (constantly!) throws his boxers onto the bathroom floor before he gets into the shower, and somehow *doesn't see them anymore* when he gets back out. Boxers, what boxers? Sigh . . . (I think I need some chocolate.)

Instead, maybe you'll appreciate him more too—and your children, and your friends, and even the work you have to do. Because it's all part of your beautiful life—your life that is filled with special moments.

When you view life with more gratitude and avoid your inner snide side (I know I have one!), you truly do start to appreciate the little things more. The simple act of kindness to yourself—your sweet moment—can expand to become little acts of kindness to others.

One of my favorite once-in-a-while sweets is a piece of Vosges chocolate (www.vosgeschocolate.com), a company in Chicago that makes chocolates like nothing you've ever eaten before. Their truffles are true works of art and their bars are taste sensations—some are flavored with hot peppers or Indian spices, or even bacon! It's a party in your mouth.

Sometimes I buy a big eight-dollar bar and break off one square a day. It lasts for over a week. The key is to savor it slowly and with deep appreciation. You know . . . like when your husband finds *your* sweet spot.

One of my neighbors is the youngest eighty-two-year-old I've ever encountered. She looks and moves like a person decades younger than she is. When I asked her what her secret was, she said, "A bit of chocolate every day." To me, this is just further proof of what I already know—that a brownie from the local bakery cut into bite-size pieces or a little chocolate-chip cookie or a piece of really great chocolate is exactly what we all need to live a long, healthy, happy, contented life.

Maybe I'll have a slice of toast with a teaspoon of Nutella (a chocolate hazelnut paste . . . peanut butter's sexy cousin!), or a smoothie made of peanut butter, chocolate, and bananas. Once you get your mind around the concept of savoring a small amount rather than mindlessly stuffing in a large amount, sugar takes on a whole new life.

4. TRY JUICING. I'LL GET YOU STARTED.

Real Moms know that eating fresh, concentrated juices from fruits and vegetables can boost your energy in the most wonderful ways. Juicing is an easy, inexpensive way to do this, and it's fun, too. If you don't already have one, go shopping for a juicer. You can spend a lot or a little. I recommend looking for the easiest one to clean. Then let your kids help push those chunks of fresh fruits and veggies into the juicer (no fingers, please—use the food-pushing tool!). When juicing, use organic local fruits whenever you can, clean them well, and get juicy!

When I first started juicing, I went to the department store and purchased a simple and reasonably priced juicer, Jack LaLanne's Power Juicer (www.powerjuicer.com). It's just one of many good brands. When I got home, I immediately juiced apples for two days. Drink, enjoy, repeat. Then, a couple of days later, I decided to get more adventurous—I juiced apples *and* carrots. Drink, enjoy, repeat.

Later that week, I read the book *Juicing for Life: A Guide to the Health Benefits of Fresh Fruit and Vegetable Juicing*, by Cherie Calbom and Maureen Keane. That got me even more motivated to experiment with all kinds of fruits and vegetables.

I loved the idea of combining oranges (peeled) and apples, maybe adding some gingerroot juice or celery juice. The options are endless: pears, spinach, melons, carrots, grapefruit, cucumbers, pine-apples, beets, kale. (Banana and avocados don't work, FYI.) Just peel off the toughest rinds and go for it. Your mixed juices may not always be the most gorgeous colors, but they will have gorgeous tastes. Or not. Keep experimenting and finding brave new combinations of your favorite fruits and vegetables. You might even find you like the juice from some kinds of produce that you don't care for in whole form.

Drink. Enjoy. Repeat . . . a *lot*.

You don't always have to do the juicing yourself, especially not these days. As I write this, I'm battling a cold, so today while I was out, I grabbed a juice at my favorite juice bar to help supercharge my immune system. Here's what I ordered: apple-spinach-celery-carrot–green pepper–cucumber-kale juice. I'm already feeling better.

Just remember that when you juice, you remove fiber from the fruit and vegetable and you concentrate the natural sugars. It's the *essence* of the fruit or veggie, but not the whole thing, so be sure to compensate later in your day with enough fiber, such as with a bowl of whole-grain cereal or some ground flax in your smoothie or on your salad.

This week, break your juicer out of storage, or go shopping for one. Buy a bag of apples, any kind, preferably organic; a bag of carrots; a bag of celery; and a couple of other vegetables you like. If you aren't yet converted to the taste of vegetables (I haven't given up on you yet!), just add a few extra apples to keep the juice sweet.

Now fire up that juicer and start creating!

A few more juicing tips:

* To force leafy greens into the juicer, add them between chunks of apple or carrot. Because they are firmer, they will push the greens into the juicing blade. The thicker, juicier ones, like Romaine lettuce, work best.
* Cut off citrus rinds and pineapple skins, and peel mangoes and papayas before juicing.
* Once you're finished juicing, always unplug your juicer right away, disassemble it, and clean it using a dish brush and warm water. If you do it right away, the food fragments come off much more easily; trust me!

* Then kick back and enjoy your perfect, potent glass of freshly extracted juice. Drink. Enjoy. Repeat again tomorrow.

5. DRINK EIGHT GLASSES OF FRESH, PURE WATER EVERY DAY.

As you teach yourself to practice moderation, water can be your ally. After you've had your sweet treat for the day, if you feel your mouth crying out for more, have one of your eight glasses of water. It will wash your mouth clean and refocus you on the next thing, signaling that your sweet snack is over and now that you are satisfied, you can move on with your day.

So drink up!

And that's it, Real Moms. It's going to be a great week. Sweets are part of a full, healthy life of normal eating that also includes family time, playtime, outside time in the sunlight and fresh air, nourishing meals, and enthusiasm for the pleasure in life. It's not *all* about the sugar.

Enjoying sweets is all about *balance*. Fill up your desserts with high-quality ingredients, love, and a sense of fun, and you and your children will learn to live lives full of pleasure instead of guilt.

Sweet!

PART TWO

Getting Serious:

Making the
Real Moms Love to Eat Plan
Part of Your Life

WEEK SEVEN:

Do It in the Kitchen

THIS WEEK, DO FIVE THINGS:

1. Organize your kitchen. Get rid of anything you don't use regularly. Go for *clean*.
2. Upgrade one nonstick pan in your kitchen with one stainless-steel or cast-iron pan. Practice using it. I'll give you some tips.
3. Tackle those plastic storage containers. Clear them out and replace them with glass ones. I'll show you the easiest and most economical way to do this.
4. Read the label, Mabel. What are the stats, bottom line? Can you toss it?
5. Are you still drinking your eight glasses of fresh, pure water every day? Out of a BPA-free container?

N EVERY MEANINGFUL love affair, there comes a point when you have to admit that either it's not going to work out or you've moved beyond flirtation and you're starting to get serious. I mean *serious*, serious. I mean the c-word: *committed*.

Up to this point, the Real Moms Love to Eat plan has been a lot of fun—you've been going on "dates" with exotic new fruits and vegetables, having exciting new experiences with juicers and Vitamixes and spiralizers, indulging in a little afternoon delight with the dark chocolate of your choice. And I'm guessing you're feeling pretty good. Giddy, even. Sexier.

Wouldn't you like to feel like this *all the time?*

You can. You just have to step up to the plate and commit to your new lifestyle of pleasure and health. It's time to take things to the next level—to go beyond flirting and dating and move in together. It's time to get *married* to your better, healthier relationship with food.

In this chapter, I'll help you lay the groundwork for this new level of commitment, and it all starts in your kitchen—in the way you organize it, keep it clean, care for it, and raise your standards for what you keep in there. In some ways, your kitchen is a metaphor for your body, so I want you to treat it with the same loving care and attention. You've been having a great time filling it up with better food, but now it's time to ditch the stuff that no longer serves you and go all the way. It's like throwing all that no-good cheating boyfriend's stuff onto the lawn. It's *not your problem* anymore!

I also want to have a serious heart-to-heart discussion about how to make your kitchen purer, cleaner, safer, and more environmentally friendly. It's all part of the package of pleasure and health, because when your kitchen is cleaner, it's safer, and when you cook and store food in nontoxic containers that don't harm you, your kids, or the earth, you will feel even happier, even healthier, like you're dancing more lightly on the planet.

In short, this chapter is about newlywed bliss in the kitchen.

GET ORGANIZED

Take a good hard look at your kitchen. This is where the magic begins. This is where you store the food that you and your family snack on. This is where you make the meals. This is even where you stand in front of the refrigerator and, despairing, decide it's time to order out, or go out, because you've got nothing you want to eat or cook in there. Or you just can't face the inevitable mess. Or you just don't have the energy to think about it at all. (I know. I'm a Real Mom too.)

But what if cooking and eating in your kitchen were easier, cleaner, and more fun? It can be! The first step is to get really, really organized. After all, you and your new lifestyle are moving in together. It's going to need a few drawers and some closet space . . . um, I mean, cabinet space.

When I decided to reorganize my kitchen cabinets a couple of years ago, I worked with a home organizer named Molly. This was such a worthwhile expense! She showed me how to create flow in my kitchen. Doesn't that sound nice? *Flow.* It's what every functional kitchen needs.

The first thing we did was to pull everything out of every single cabinet and drawer. This might sound overwhelming, but it was an essential step, because if I hadn't taken it all out, most of it would have stayed in there, and that includes a lot of junk I didn't need. Molly helped me to evaluate every single thing and decide what I really needed and used, and what I didn't even remember I had! We separated everything into three piles: "Keep," "Donate," and "Not Sure." We also kept a big trash bag handy. Out went the tomato-sauce-stained old plastic food-storage containers. Out went all the overused, scratched-up plastic cups. Out went everything broken, chipped, or too worn-out to be useful. Anything that had somehow sneaked into the kitchen that really belonged somewhere else went back to "somewhere else." When I had too much of something—I found I had three spatulas—I donated one and just kept two. It took several hours, but it was so liberating to clear the clutter and make room for the small appliances that can actually make my meal prep easier.

Next, we returned everything to the cabinets and drawers, but in an organized fashion, with a plan. We added inserts (like small plastic containers or mini boxes) to help separate items so I could find things when I needed them. We set aside a big red toolbox for all the excess tools I use sometimes but not often, to keep them out of the way, so they wouldn't clutter up my cabinets. Then we added cabinet shelf extenders to make more storage.

In the pantry, we organized and categorized all the food and paper products and large platters so I could get to everything I needed. By having all the food categorized, I could keep a better inventory for future shopping trips. We installed a shopping list in the pantry, complete with a pencil, so I could keep a running list of what to buy for the week. No more forgetting something crucial, or accidentally buying something I already have.

One of my favorite things we did was to put a lazy Susan in the middle of the kitchen table, stocked with sea salt, black pepper, and herbal seasonings. When it's sitting right there in front of you, you *will* use it.

Cleaning and organizing my kitchen in this way almost made me feel like I had a completely remodeled kitchen! It felt airier and cleaner, and I could find everything without knocking things over to get to what I needed.

Although I'm really glad I hired an organizer, you don't actually need one to make over your kitchen in this way. Just take an afternoon, pull everything out of your kitchen, and be ruthless about what you put back in. Get rid of the old, scratched, stained, dented cookware, storage containers, and serving pieces. Most people have more of this stuff than they ever use. Got multiple sets of dishes? Donate some. Sentiment is nice if you've got the space for it, but if you don't, you'll feel so much lighter and cleaner and calmer in your kitchen if you clear out the junk.

Put back only what you actually need. If you use it every week or more often, put it where it's easy to grab. If you want to use it more because it's in line with your new healthier lifestyle (the juicer, the mandoline, the food processor), make it more accessible. If you use it less than once a week, stow it somewhere out of the way, so you can get it when you need it but it won't be blocking the more useful items. If you haven't used it in a year and it doesn't have any great sentimental value, I suggest getting rid of it. You might want to keep Grandma's antique china, but that set of stoneware you got at a garage sale when you were first married that you haven't touched in five years? Is it really worth the kitchen real estate it's taking up?

And if it's not something in line with what you're doing now (do you really need to deep-fat-fry your Thanksgiving turkey? How badly do you need a doughnut maker?), maybe it's time to part ways.

For me, a big priority for getting rid of something also had to do with toxicity. So let's talk about *that*.

PURIFY YOUR POTS AND PANS

Let's talk chemicals. This is an area of great concern to me. Before I had children, I never gave my cookware or storage containers or even my water bottle a second thought. I would make my omelets or grilled cheese sandwiches in my nonstick pan. I would store my leftovers and even reheat them in plastic containers. I would swill my daily H_2O from a plastic one-liter bottle. It was all easy, and easy to clean. Easy is good, right?

But when I was pregnant and decided to make my home as clean and safe as I could, I started doing some research and I was amazed at what I learned.

First, let's consider your pots and pans. Most people own heavy-weight aluminum cookware coated with a nonstick or anodized aluminum coating. These kinds of pots and pans are relatively inexpensive, and they are very good heat conductors, so they give you reliable results. However, when nonstick pans are heated to a high temperature, used a lot, washed in a dishwasher or with an abrasive cleaner, or scarred by sharp scrubbers or metal utensils like spatulas and tongs, that nonstick coating begins to chip, peel away, and break down . . . right into your food.

In fact, according to the Environmental Working Group (EWG), cookware coated with nonstick coating such as Teflon can, on a conventional cooktop, quickly exceed the temperature at which the coating breaks apart and emits toxic particles and also toxic gases. These gases have been linked to hundreds and perhaps thousands of pet bird deaths. It's the canary-in-the-coal-mine effect—the smallest, most sensitive creatures with the most delicate respiratory systems are the first to go.

But what is this nonstick coating doing to humans, especially children? Many people believe these fumes and particles may also be linked to an unknown number of human illnesses and chronic conditions. In an EWG study conducted by a university food-safety professor, a general nonstick frying pan was put onto a conventional electric stovetop. It reached a temperature of 736 degrees Fahrenheit in three minutes, twenty seconds, and a Teflon-coated pan reached 721 degrees Fahrenheit in five minutes under the same conditions. According to DuPont, which makes Teflon, Teflon "off-gases toxic particulates" at 464 degrees Fahrenheit, and at 680 degrees Fahrenheit, the Teflon pans release at least six toxic gases. Some of these toxic gases are carcinogenic, some are known global pollutants, some are known to be lethal to humans in low doses, and one is a known chemical warfare agent and an analog of nerve gas.

Um . . . yikes?

DuPont maintains that their pans do not decompose significantly at temperatures below 660 degrees Fahrenheit, and that normal cooking does not reach these temperatures, but the EWG studies proved otherwise. Meanwhile, the Environmental Protection Agency enlisted a panel of experts to study the use of a chemical called PFOA, a common component of Teflon, and most members of the panel agreed at the conclusion of the study that the substance was a "likely human carcinogen."

When birds suffer from Teflon toxicosis, their lungs hemorrhage and fill with fluid, suffocating them. But nobody, including the government, has studied the possible health effects on humans. When humans suffer from exposure to these fumes, it's called polymer fume fever, and it is characterized by flulike symptoms, from headache, chills, sore throat, and fever to shortness of breath, tightness in the chest, and malaise. According to some studies, 95 percent of Americans have detectible levels of Teflon-related chemicals in their blood. Even if they have no symptoms . . . yet . . . it all sounds pretty scary to me. Not everybody agrees that these nonstick chemicals are hazardous, but nobody has proved they are safe.

I don't know about you, but I'd rather not wait around for the government to send me an official notice that toxic fumes and particulate matter from my kitchen might be harming my babies. Call me an alarmist if you want to, but I prefer to live by the "better safe than sorry" motto when it comes to something like this. I may be petite, but I'm a grizzly bear when it comes to protecting my kids, and I know you are too. It's biological. It's nature.

Nonstick coating, on the other hand, has nothing to do with nature. In fact, I would even call it an aberration of nature, especially when it is applied to the surface of a vessel in which we prepare the food we then put into our bodies, and into the bodies of our little ones.

"Tell us how you really feel, Beth!"

Oh, you know I will.

So here's my advice, which you can take or leave, according to your inclinations, your budget, and your beliefs: Throw the nonstick stuff into the trash! Don't even donate it, because you're just passing along a health hazard to someone else and her children.

So what are your options? You may be wondering, as you dangle your heretofore trustworthy nonstick skillet over the gaping maw of the garbage can, how the heck you are going to cook tomorrow morning's scrambled eggs, or grilled cheese sandwiches, or stir-fries.

Real Moms have options! Other types of cookware may not be as familiar to you, but they are safer and perfectly easy to use once you get the hang of them. Let's have a cookware meet-and-greet.

CAST IRON: Cast-iron pans are heavy but, boy, are they great. You can use them on any heat source and they can go from stove to oven without worry (although you might need both hands to lift one). When you first buy or inherit one, season it by coating the inside with oil and heating it gently on the stove, then letting it cool. Never use soap on it, but every time you use it, scrub it out with water and a scrubber (and a bit of salt if you need a more abrasive agent), dry it, and coat it with a little more oil. It will soon develop a coating just as good as nonstick, but totally safe. Your scrambled eggs should come out just fine, and your parakeet need not cower in fear.

You'll find higher-end cast-iron pans coated in ceramic, as with the Le Creuset brand of cookware from France. These also resist sticking and they last forever. Plus, they have cool old-school cookware shapes, like big soup pots with heavy lids and round or oval "French ovens" (or Dutch ovens) as well as griddles and bakeware.

STAINLESS STEEL: People tend to be scared off by stainless-steel cookware, maybe because of a bad experience with sticking food. However, stainless steel has many advantages. Not only is it nontoxic, not only can you use your metal spatula, not only can it go from stove to oven (as long as the handles are also ovenproof), but you can *put it in the dishwasher*! This alone is a big plus in my book.

As for stainless steel's bad reputation for hanging on to food and never letting go, food *will* stick if you put it in the pan cold. However, if you heat up your stainless-steel pan so it's nice and hot, then add the oil or butter just before adding the food, you won't have a mess, except for the natural residue from browning, which makes a great sauce. Just remove your meat or vegetables after they've cooked, pour in a splash of wine or broth to "deglaze" the pan, and scrub away with your wooden spoon or spatula to dislodge all those yummy browned bits. A dash of salt, a pinch of pepper, maybe a teaspoon of butter mixed in, and you've got a sauce worthy of a French chef. Ooh-la-la!

With stainless steel, thicker is better. Thin pans do tend to burn and stick more. You don't need to buy a whole set, though. Just buy the pieces you really use, like one good skillet with a lid and one good saucepan with a lid. Do you ever really use anything else?

Once you get over your dependency on nonstick, a whole new culinary world will open up, and if you're like me, you'll feel so much better knowing you've got those volatile toxins out of your home.

CERAMIC: Ceramic bakeware or stoneware is a great option for casseroles, cakes, even cookie sheets. CorningWare is one of the oldest—I still remember the little blue flowers on my mother's CorningWare pan. For pots and pans, I like Mercola cookware—they make not just pots, pans, and utensils for cooking, but bakeware and all the accessories you need to make a nice, nontoxic pot of tea. Pampered Chef makes a line of ceramic bakeware, including muffin tins, cake pans, pie plates, and cookie sheets. My absolute favorite, however, is Emile Henry—from cassoulet pots to pie dishes to matching spice jars, this French-made line of cookware is gorgeous and amazingly easy to clean after soaking in hot water. *Oui!*

GLASS: Glass is a renewable resource, and it works especially well for baking casseroles and pies, as long as you reduce your oven temperature by 25 degrees when baking (glass saves on energy!).

While I remember glass saucepans back in the 1970s, I also remember that they weren't ideal for the stovetop. Maybe that's why they don't make them anymore.

The Old Bamboo

THE LATEST IN environmentally friendly kitchens includes fast-growing, sustainable, renewable bamboo. The material makes great cutting boards, cheese boards, "wooden" spoons, tongs, and spatulas, and it can also be used for kitchen backsplashes and flooring. Consider using a bamboo steamer and paddles for your steamed vegetables, as bamboo is a totally nonreactive material that is fortunately modestly priced. The texture of the bamboo allows steam to circulate and evaporate so that less moisture will form on the inside of the lid. Clean, lean veggies in a snap!

PARE DOWN THE PLASTIC

But wait! Just when you thought it was safe to eat in your kitchen . . . and that I had come down from my soapbox . . . what about those plastic storage containers?

Plastic containers are cheap, convenient, lightweight, even disposable. Aren't they perfect for holding your leftovers until tomorrow, or for packing in your kids' lunch boxes? Or for your *infant's formula*?

Recently, public health and consumer groups reported that when baby bottles were heated, the plastic released a hormone-disrupting chemical called Bisphenol A, or BPA. It's a compound in hard, clear, polycarbonate plastic, and the scientific consensus seems to be that yes, it will leach into your water, or whatever else it holds. BPA has been shown to mimic the effects of estrogen and interfere with hormone levels, even increasing the risk of uterine fibroids, breast cancer, decreased sperm count, and prostate cancer. Some studies also show that BPA in plastic mouse cages harmed the development of mouse eggs, and that BPA in the environment could even damage an unborn baby's growth. Of course, sensitive babies and young children (clutching their plastic sippy cups) are at the greatest risk because of their young, developing systems.

Another study out of the University of Cincinnati reported evidence that BPA can actually disrupt the developing brain. One of the study's lead scientists, Scott Belcher, PhD, associate professor of pharmacology and cell biophysics and corresponding study author, stated: "While plastics are typically thought of as being stable, scientists have known for many years that the chemical linkage between BPA molecules was unstable, and that BPA leaches into food or beverages in contact with the plastics."

Baby bottles, in particular, leach BPA into formula, breast milk, juice, or any other liquid, and the older the bottle, the more it leaches. As I write this, legal battles are ongoing about banning plastics containing BPA, and California lawmakers just rejected a ban on BPA in baby bottles, sippy cups, and infant formula cans. Usage has already been cut dramatically in Europe, but the United States seems to be resistant to limiting the chemical in its cheap plastic products. While they fight it out, maybe you want to think twice about popping that plastic container of macaroni and cheese into the microwave, or filling up that old baby bottle again?

There are ways to tell whether your plastic containers contain BPA. BPA-free plastics include polyethylene (marked with the number 2 in the recycling triangle on the bottom of the container), and polypropylene plastic (marked with recycling number 5). The other numbers contain BPA.

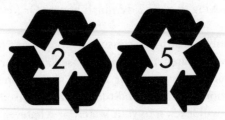

However, I have an even better solution, just in case those plastics eventually reveal some other hazardous component: Skip it altogether. Use glass.

Several years ago, I replaced all my plastic containers with inexpensive, sturdy, safe Pyrex containers. You can find glass storage containers in various sizes at any supermarket or kitchen store. I also like the glass storage solutions from Crate & Barrel, with BPA-free plastic lids.

I love knowing glass is nonreactive and won't add chemicals to my kids' food, but I also appreciate their aesthetic appeal. They just look nicer, and the food is so easy to see. No more peeking into the plastic mystery box wondering what you put in there last week. Glass is clear as day.

You don't have to spend any money, either. Every time you buy a jar of salsa or spaghetti sauce or pickles or artichoke hearts, just run the glass container through the dishwasher and then use it for storing leftovers. Free storage containers!

I also avoid serving food in plastic (and especially heating it up in plastic!). Serve in glass or use recycled paper plates if you really need something nonbreakable and/or disposable. I like the Eco-Forward® line of Bare by Solo, which is durable, recyclable, and made from sustainable materials (www.barebysolo.com). For disposable elegance, try VerTerra disposable plates, made from fallen palm leaves; they are gorgeous and you can throw them in the compost pile. Find a store that carries them on their Web site at www.VerTerra.com.

And while you might not want to let your toddler carry a glass bottle around the house, you can certainly feed your infant out of one. If nothing else, make sure all the baby bottles and sippy cups in your house are made from BPA-free plastic.

Canned!

WORRIED ABOUT BPA? Me too! If you are, you should know that it sometimes hides in the unlikeliest places. The linings of metal food cans often contain BPA. According to several studies, BPA has been found in the linings of cans of peas, artichokes, beans, mixed vegetables, corn, and mushrooms. When possible, buy your food packed in glass instead of a can.

Ahh . . . now, doesn't your kitchen feel cleaner and clearer and nicer already? Don't you just want to go in there and cook something? Yeah, about that . . . as long as you are making over your cooking tools, you might as well go all the way. Let's take a look at the food.

Imagine, if you will, a beautiful ripe red apple dangling from an apple tree. It's juicy. It's ready to pick and eat. So, what's on its ingredient list?

Ingredient list, you ask? What ingredient list? It's an apple. It contains . . . *apple.*

Exactly.

We've all got some packaged food in the house. It's practically impossible to avoid, unless you want to live a totally Spartan existence and you have nothing else to do all day but grind your own wheat and bake your own bread and go outside to slaughter your own chickens. Even some of the simplest foods we are used to eating come in packages—a loaf of bread, a jar of peanut butter, a bag of salad; even flour, sugar, and yeast come in packages unless you buy them in bulk at a health food store (and then you have to bring your own package to get them home).

It's the twenty-first century, and as nice as it sounds, it's just not reasonable to say you shouldn't eat any packaged food.

However . . .

I teach grade-school children a program called Nutrition Detectives, designed by some of my teachers from the Institute of Integrative Nutrition (Drs. David and Catherine Katz). This educational program emphasizes the importance of making healthy choices while eating, and if it was just a matter of saying, "Don't eat food in a package," I'm not sure it would go over so well with the grade-school crowd. Instead, the program teaches children how to read food labels, detect deceptive marketing practices, and learn how to identify and subsequently choose the healthiest foods.

It gets kids in on the secret, enlisting them to be supermarket detectives. And it points kids not to the "nutrition information box," with its cryptic percentages, but to the ingredient list, where they can actually see what's in that neon-colored fruit snack or snack cake or bag of crunchy chips or box of cereal. Then *they* get to decide: Take it, or *leave it?*

To make this very clear for kids, we talk about "'no' foods." These are the ingredients that are not good for kids (or *you*) and that are best avoided:

* Sugars (including high-fructose corn syrup or corn sugar)
* Partially hydrogenated fats (known as trans fats)
* Processed grains (typically flour)

It's not that you can't ever, *ever* eat them. It's just that you really should think twice, and maybe you'll choose to say, *Thanks, but no, thanks.*

Maybe you'll choose to *leave it.* If little kids can get this, it'll be a cinch for a Real Mom like you. Oftentimes, when adults approach things more simply, like a child, things become clearer. A kid-friendly approach never hurt anybody.

My friend Jane and I were talking one day and we realized that, growing up, both of us used to eat Lucky Charms—which has not lost quite all of its charm for her, though she has grown into an adventurous and health-conscious eater. Jane had found an alternative to our mutual childhood mania for the magically delicious breakfast "charms," from a company called Three Sisters: Marshmallow Oaties, a sweetened, whole-grain, toasted-oat cereal with marshmallows and no artificial flavors or colors.

That means instead of yellow #5 and #6, red #40, and blue #1, you get blueberry, pumpkin, and carrot concentrates for color. It's an improvement. And it's a good first step in upping the quality of the food in your kitchen—even when it does come in a package.

Fortunately, Marshmallow Oaties are not an anomaly. You can walk the aisles of any health food store, like Trader Joe's, Whole Foods Market, Sprouts, or your local food co-op (and, increasingly, even the natural foods aisle in your local supermarket) and find hundreds of healthy "snack food" alternatives free of dyes, chemicals, saturated fats, or preservatives. You can buy natural versions of other cereals, toaster pastries, flavored oatmeal packets, fruit snacks, and even candy. You can also find chips, crackers, chicken (or vegetarian "chicken") nuggets, frozen dinners, and dessert in just about any incarnation, all free of the standard chemical preservatives and artificial colors and flavors of conventional junk food. No, it's not perfect food. No, it's not whole food. But it is a step in the right direction, getting the chemicals out and the good stuff in. Baby steps!

Of course, you won't know the good from the bad unless you *read the label*, so let me just emphasize that point again. It's all on the package—the government requires it. Don't look at the health claims on the front. Look at the ingredient list. Is it natural? Organic? Whole-grain? Free of trans fats and HFCS and artificial ingredients?

The next step is to shoot for foods with fewer ingredients. The ideal would be to shoot for whole foods or packaged foods with fewer than five ingredients, whether they are for your kids or for your own snacking pleasure. Let's go back to that cereal. Just this afternoon, I snacked on a bowl of regular old-fashioned oats with sliced strawberries, walnuts, wheat germ, and rice milk. (Wheat germ is processed to separate the germ from the rest of the kernel, and rice milk has several ingredients aside from water, rice, and a bit of oil . . . but not too long a list.) It was good food.

I know how it is—it's so much easier and faster to open a package of something than to make it yourself, but really, how hard was it for me to eat oats with fruit and nuts? It didn't take much more time than opening the cereal box. There are so many ways you can do this every day. What do you crave? What are the kids clamoring for? Before mindlessly tearing open a package, just stop and think for a minute—how quickly could you make it yourself? Mix nuts, pretzels, dried fruit, and chocolate chips together for homemade trail mix. Slice up whole-grain tortillas and bake them for homemade chips—or bake potato chips by thinly slicing potatoes, brushing them with canola oil, and baking them at 400 degrees until crispy. No ingredients list involved. Try some of the dehydrated cracker recipes in this book, on pages 95–96. Or just have some fruit, vegetables, peanut butter, low-fat cheese. . . .

I know you won't always have time to make your snacks at home, and sometimes nothing satisfies like a bag of chips or a package of cookies. But here's the point: To do what's right by your own body and for your family, take a good hard look at the processed food in your cabinets. Can you eat it less often? Can you make something yourself a little more often? Can you make the healthier choice most of the time? And as for the packages themselves, what deserves to stay?

And what deserves the boot?

DO FIVE THINGS

You don't have to spend thousands of dollars remodeling your kitchen. This week, keep it simple and take some first steps to a more committed relationship to feeling and looking great. Just do these five things to make over your kitchen, and you'll feel like a new woman.

1. ORGANIZE YOUR KITCHEN. GET RID OF ANYTHING YOU DON'T USE REGULARLY. GO FOR *CLEAN*.

Take a morning or an afternoon or even a weekend. Pull everything out of that kitchen. Toss the junk. Give away the stuff you don't use. *Don't put it back into the kitchen unless you know you actually will use it!*

2. UPGRADE ONE NONSTICK PAN IN YOUR KITCHEN TO ONE STAINLESS-STEEL OR CAST-IRON PAN. PRACTICE USING IT.

It's scratched and getting old anyway, isn't it? If you can't bear to ditch all your nonstick cookware, this week at least get rid of your very worst nonstick pan. Just throw it straight into the trash. Now, get to know cast iron or stainless steel. Wash it well. If it's cast iron, season it by oiling the inside well and heating it, then letting it cool.

Then use it! Heat it up, add some oil, and sauté something yummy, like sliced potatoes with sea salt and pepper, or chicken with green peppers and onions, or turkey burgers. Notice how it works compared to your old pan.

3. TACKLE THOSE PLASTIC STORAGE CONTAINERS. CLEAR THEM OUT AND REPLACE THEM WITH GLASS ONES.

Ditch 'em all, or just the worst ones, with the stains and scratches or the missing lids. All at once or piece by piece, commit to replacing them with glass.

4. READ THE LABEL, MABEL. WHAT ARE THE STATS, BOTTOM LINE? CAN YOU TOSS IT?

Get into that pantry, that refrigerator, that cupboard. Throw out the junk. Just do it. It's time. (But leave the stuff you really love . . . like the dark chocolate!)

5. ARE YOU STILL DRINKING YOUR EIGHT GLASSES OF FRESH, PURE WATER EVERY DAY? OUT OF A BPA-FREE CONTAINER?

Water is the key to energy. Have you noticed, as you've been drinking more water these past few weeks, that you feel more energetic? It's easy to mistake signals of dehydration for hunger, but eating won't solve the problem. Dehydration can also lead to loss of appetite, dry skin, dry mouth, chills, muscle cramps, fatigue, or even head rushes. By the time you feel thirsty, you are already starting to get dehydrated.

Instead, pay attention to the color of your urine. If it's very pale, almost clear, you're probably well hydrated. If it's very yellow, most likely you are dehydrated.

As a mother it's also important that you monitor your child's water intake daily. Don't force it on them, but make sure your kids drink some water every day, at least a few good glasses. A simple equation for adults and children alike is to take their weight and divide it in half; the number you get is the number in ounces of water. So a hundred-and-twenty-pound person would drink approximately sixty ounces of clear water (not mixed in tea, juices, or soups) daily.

Dehydration symptoms in children may include irritability, tiredness, or lack of concentration. Water is an essential element in neurological transmission, and poor hydration could adversely affect a child's mental performance and learning ability. Teach your kids to pay attention to their urine too throughout the day. (Just don't tell them this in front of their friends—how embarrassing!) If it's getting dark yellow, make sure they know to have another glass of water. (And no, soda doesn't count.)

Wow, I feel cleaner already, just *talking* about purging the toxins and junk from Real Mom kitchens everywhere! I hope you do too. And now that your kitchen is so ready, clean, clear, pure, spacious, and welcoming, it's time to get in there and get busy.

CHAPTER
EIGHT

WEEK EIGHT:

Commit to Whole Foods

THIS WEEK, DO FIVE THINGS:

1. Expand your produce repertoire. Find a new fruit or vegetable you've never tried, learn how to prepare it, and give it a try.
2. Precut vegetables for salads or snacks at the beginning of the week, and keep them fresh with some tricks that I'll show you.
3. Cook once; eat two or even three times. I'll show you how.
4. Call in the reinforcements! Why should you have to do it all alone? I'll show you how to delegate easy kitchen jobs for kids of all ages . . . and even husbands. Plus, my secret motivational strategies for getting kids excited about cooking.
5. I know you are still drinking your eight glasses of fresh, pure water every day. Is it a habit yet?

WITH YOUR NEW all-that kitchen and your new all-that attitude, you're probably feeling pretty darned good about your new level of commitment to your new all-that lifestyle. You are *so over* the junk that makes you feel less than your best, sexiest self.

But then . . . you have to start cooking and eating without the junk. And the junk was easy. And fun. And cheap. Like that exboyfriend you *know* was bad for you, but, well . . . he was a really good kisser!

I know what you're thinking. You're thinking that you loved the *idea* of getting healthy and strong and feeding your family the best foods possible, but what you didn't totally recognize was that a full-on commitment to healthy living actually takes some *work*.

Is the honeymoon really over?

Real Moms know perfectly well that every meaningful relationship takes some work, but that the benefits actually are worth the effort. The great news about the Real Moms Love to Eat plan is that the benefits begin *ASAP* . . . as in *right now*.

Besides, the whole point of hanging out with other Real Moms is to get you through these tough times when you just can't bear the thought of chopping vegetables, and the pizza delivery guy is haunting your dreams with his siren song of cheap pepperoni and melted cheese.

So let's have a quick reality check. *Nobody said you can't ever order another pizza!* Nobody said you can't have potato chips when you want them, or some packaged cookies, or even the occasional (gasp!) toaster pastry or (shriek!) packaged snack cake. It's true: Those aren't snacks that will make you feel good if you eat them on a daily basis, but Real Moms aren't about extremes. We simply don't have the time. Or, I should say, we have more important things to do with our time, like snuggle or play with the kids, walk the dog, enjoy a romantic glass of wine with our husbands, or just *enjoy dinner*.

So let go of the stress.

Instead, this chapter is about helping you enjoy and relish and even *love* to prepare real, fresh, whole foods—even if it does involve just a teensy bit of vegetable chopping.

WHOLE FOOD LOVE

Let's talk about food. *Real* food. *Whole* food. Food the way nature made it, not a factory. Whole food is the *key*, ladies. I mean it when I say this, with all my heart. Whole food is the secret element that will allow you to savor and indulge in and love food without overeating. Whole food is filling, natural, and your body understands what it is. It hasn't had anything stripped away from it, so it contains all the elements nature intended to fill you up and nourish you.

But remember, we're not about extremes. As long as you are eating about 80 percent whole food, the other 20 percent can consist of all the yummy foods you love that just happen to be a little more processed than, say, an apple or a salad. No guilt! Have what you want—and nourish yourself with mostly whole food. Now all you have to do is learn how to prepare it so it's absolutely irresistible.

One of the great things about what you are doing with the Real Moms Love to Eat plan is that you are getting your children used to whole foods. They are forming habits that will last them a lifetime, thanks to you. (You are *such* a good mom!) But the great thing about discovering and investing in whole foods as an *adult* is that you finally have the palate to really appreciate them.

Maybe you think you're a picky eater and maybe you don't, but the simple fact is that mature palates can tolerate and even learn to love foods that might have been too strong or unusual-tasting to a younger you. Plus, as you get older and more experienced and you learn more about food, you might discover and be adventurous enough to try new foods you never even noticed in the market before. Add to that the simple fact that most supermarkets and grocery stores are responding to the twenty-first-century consumer's desire for more variety.

All these factors come together to result in so many delicious new foods that are available to you now.

So let's think about the foods that you might typically overlook in the market. For me, the stars of late have been pomegranates, parsnips, kale, and red cabbage. These nutritional stars are all whole foods, and now that I've tried them, they've become a regular part of my diet.

So pardon me while I wax poetic for a moment.

What could be sexier than a pomegranate? Round and full and rosy, these hard-shelled fruits are filled with juicy little ruby-colored seeds so full of flavor, you'll swear they're sinful. In fact, pomegranates are the stuff of myths—when Hades stole the beautiful Persephone and carried her down to the underworld, she was allowed to return only if she didn't eat anything. But she did eat something—Hades, the king of the underworld, persuaded her to eat just a handful of pomegranate seeds. This decadent dietary infraction got her six months in hell every year—the cause, according to the Greek myth, of winter. When Persephone returns to earth each year, spring arrives.

Lucky for you, pomegranates won't land you in hell. In fact, they'll send you straight to heaven when you taste their bursting, juicy flavor. Aside from being an exotic, gorgeous treat for which I often get a hankering (especially around the winter holidays, when they are abundant), pomegranates are high in vitamin C and a good source of vitamin B6, potassium, and antioxidants. The tiny seed inside the aril provides crunch, fiber, and micronutrients.

Pomegranates 101

POMEGRANATES ROCK—BUT HOW the heck do you eat one? If you don't know what to do with a pomegranate, it can be downright puzzling. But you're a whole-foods ace now, so it's time to step up and claim power over the pomegranate! Here's what to do:

1. Cut your pomegranate in half, then in quarters.
2. Stretch open the pieces so you can easily roll the juicy seed casings (called arils) free of the pith with your fingers. Or immerse them in a bowl of water and work the seeds free from the white pith. The seeds will sink and the pith will float, and you'll contain the inevitable crimson tide of sweet, delicious juice.
3. Pour off or otherwise discard the pith, drain the seeds in a strainer if using the bowl-of-water method, and stir them into yogurt, decorate your bowl of cut fruit, or just pop them like candy. Because they *are* like candy—but sexier.

But fruits are easy to love. What about the more humble vegetable? What about a vegetable you've probably heard about but may never have actually tasted or included in your own cooking? What about parsnips?

Parsnips look like white carrots; they're closely related, but parsnips require peeling and cooking before eating, and they are higher in vitamins and minerals (especially potassium) than their carrot brethren. Winter is peak parsnip season, and a perfect time to prepare them. Roasting coaxes the tough and reticent parsnip to soften up and become downright charming—sweet, tender, and a little nutty (like your favorite cousin?).

Parsnip Perfection

ONE EASY FAVORITE meal of mine is to fill a baking pan (about nine by thirteen inches, or the size you would use to make a lasagna) full of vegetables cut into ½-inch cubes. I especially like to use root vegetables for this recipe, such as parsnips, carrots, potatoes, beets, and/or turnips (another off-the-beaten-path veggie you should try if you don't already love them). I might add other vegetables I happen to have in the vegetable crisper, such as mushrooms, onions, peeled garlic cloves, and winter or summer squash, so the vegetables make more or less a single layer. Toss with olive oil so the veggies are lightly coated; add salt, pepper, and any other spices you like (such as cumin or chili powder); then roast for thirty to forty minutes in a preheated 400-degree oven, stirring occasionally. This is an excellent way to entice your children to enjoy their vegetables. They are practically french fries!

Another simple way to include parsnips in your diet is in miso soup, the fastest homemade soup to whip up that I know. Miso—a paste made of fermented rice, barley, or soybeans—is a living food that makes instant vegetable stock, and the paste will keep in your refrigerator for a year or more. Here's one of my favorite fifteen-minute meals: Bring a few cups of water to boil, along with chopped veggies of any sort, such as parsnips, carrots, onions, and leafy greens. Lower the heat and simmer for ten to fifteen minutes, or until the veggies are cooked to your liking. Turn off the heat and add a

(continued)

heaping tablespoon of miso for every cup of water, and stir until the miso is completely dissolved. There you have it—"instant" soup that you can feel good about serving your family. (For a raw-food version, don't boil the veggies. Just warm up water to a near boil, turn off the heat, add miso and raw veggies, and enjoy!)

Kale is another star in my list of top-favorite "adult palate" foods. When I was a little girl, I wasn't saving my allowance to buy kale at the corner store, it's true, but now I love the stuff, not just because of how nutritious it is (and it is—kale offers an abundant supply of vitamin C, beta carotene, iron, calcium, and other essential nutrients). Kale tastes delish. It comes in several varieties and ranges in taste from slightly spicy to mildly nutty.

I eat steamed kale at least once a week. All I do is wash the kale, then strip the leaves from the stiff rib (the way you would strip unwanted leaves off the stem of a flower), chop the leaves into bite-size pieces, and steam for about five minutes, until the kale is tender. I eat it alone or over rice, with a bit of olive oil and umeboshi plum vinegar or lemon juice or nutritional yeast. (You can save the ribs and chop them up later to add to any homemade soup.)

Kale: Rubbed the Right Way

PEOPLE ALWAYS USED to boil or possibly sauté kale, but the new trend in kale is to eat it raw and *massaged*. Ooh, don't you love the sound of that? All you have to do is pull out the thick stems, chop up the leaves, put them in a bowl, lube them up with a splash of olive oil, add flavor with a splash of vinegar or lemon juice, cumin, a dash of cayenne, and a little salt and pepper, and then stick your hands in the bowl and rub, rub, rub the leaves between your fingers. Squeeze them. Massage them. It's sensual and weird to have your hands in the food like that, but the massaging breaks down the tough fibers and works the oil into the thick leaves to soften them. When you're finished, you'll swear that kale salad was cooked, but it's not—it's fresh, raw, tender, and tasty (see the recipe on page 209).

Finally, I have to give a nod to red cabbage. A cheap staple food in a thriftier time (wasn't it always served with meat loaf?), red cabbage may not be the most glamorous of vegetables, but don't overlook it as a tasty treat. I was visiting my friend Caren recently, and her grade-school-age daughter Clara was enthusiastically helping us make dinner by preparing the salad—her "job." But Clara is such a fan of red cabbage that our salads turned out to be 80 percent cabbage. We thought Clara's ratios were off, but it turned out we were wrong.

Red cabbage makes an excellent salad base—and entire salad, if necessary. The trick is to chop it very thinly. When I prepare it, I peel away the outer leaves, cut the head of cabbage in half, cut out the core, then start chopping with a kind of rapid stroke, using my handy, always-sharp chef's knife. If the cabbage isn't sufficiently fine (think coleslaw-fine), I further chop the pile that's accumulated on my cutting board. Red cabbage can be eaten raw or cooked. It adds color, health-supporting nutrients, and crunch to a salad.

On the rare day when my fridge is just about bare of vegetables, I usually have some part of a head of red cabbage, which is all I need to prepare an elegant gourmet salad: chopped red cabbage, olive oil, umeboshi plum vinegar (just a bit; it's very salty), and a tablespoon of gomasio—a condiment made of roasted sesame seeds, sea salt, and sometimes seaweed. Or get creative and add your favorite salad dressing, seasoning, and other vegetables, or even a handful of raw nuts or fresh or dried fruit. Scrumptious, and good raw nourishment! I know Clara prefers her colorful red-and-white salad with ranch dressing. Maybe your kids would enjoy that too.

The Beauty of a Really Great Chef's Knife

WHEN MY SECOND son was three months old, I woke up one morning and told my husband I needed to enroll in cooking school for a semester. Little did he know that this would become one of my many adventures on my journey to becoming a Real Mom Who Loves to Eat!

So I signed up and got all geared up with my "official" white chef's hat, jacket, and black-and-white plaid pants. I donned my

(continued)

steel-toed shoes for kitchen safety and I padded off to the Cooking and Hospitality Institute of Chicago (which is now known as Le Cordon Bleu Chicago). I felt so *professional*. Once a week, I studied in the professional chef's program.

I learned more about cooking and the kitchen in that semester than I had my entire life, but one of the most important things I learned was that the uniform is one thing, but what really makes a chef is *knife skills*, and before you can learn how to wield a chef's knife properly, you have to have a proper chef's knife.

Every Real Mom must decide for herself which chef's knife feels right in her hands. The knife should be high-quality, and it should feel good in your hand—well balanced and easy to use. Your hand shouldn't slip or tire using it. Some people prefer a lighter knife, and some a heavier knife. There are many good brands, but after test-driving several, I discovered that Wüsthof was my favorite. Any good kitchen store should have a variety of high-quality chef's knives for you to try. When purchasing one, also spring for a sharpener of some kind. Even the best knives need regular sharpening to perform at the level a professional chef . . . or a Real Mom . . . demands!

BUT . . . SERIOUSLY. WHOLE FOODS? WHO HAS THE TIME?

I hear you, Real Moms! I do. Sometimes I have so much to do, I contemplate whether I really need to sleep (of course, my answer is always: *Yes, you need to sleep!*). So as much as I love my chef's knife, I get that you aren't all that crazy about spending an extra hour every evening chopping vegetables just because it's supposedly going to make you feel more energetic. It's an hour chopping vegetables. Isn't that the point of processed food—they do all that processing *for you*? Is a little extra energy really worth all that trouble? (Of course, my answer is always, *Yes, it is worth all that trouble!* But don't worry; I know how to compromise.)

Why is it that whenever we eat a salad out at a restaurant or someone else makes it for us, it tastes so much better? Because someone else made it for us, that's why. It's always nice to have someone else do all the work and then serve the food right to you, but think about this: It's also nice to eat food that hasn't been touched by people you don't know, and that hasn't had who knows what added into it!

There are many ways to make whole foods at home more efficiently and easily. I think I've tried them all. Remember the infomercials for the SaladShooter? Tried it. I've chopped my veggies in the food processor, hand chopper, spiralizer, mandoline, and any other vegetable-chopping gadget I've ever seen or even heard rumors about. I'm always searching for ways to make it just plain *easier* to have a salad.

But sometimes, in the quest to make things easier, they get more complicated.

The idea of dragging out my food processor, using it to chop a few cucumbers and carrots, and then having to clean it defeats the purpose of time well spent in the kitchen, in my opinion. Don't get me wrong; I have a real "thing" for my KitchenAid food processor, almost as if it were one of my children. I'm very protective of it, and it does many wonderful things that save me time in the kitchen, or that I couldn't easily do by hand. However, chopping vegetables isn't something that it can do more easily than I can, unless uniformity really matters or everything needs to be finely minced or pulverized.

If I actually timed the salad-making experience, I'm pretty sure the difference between using a food processor or chopper and chopping the vegetables by hand wouldn't be very much. So what's a Real Mom to do? I do have some alternative time-saving, whole-food-loving tricks that I've found most helpful.

THE SISTER-IN-LAW SOLUTION

Every time I go visit my sister-in-law, she always has such an amazing spread of food available for all of us to eat, and it always seems to be ready in a few minutes. When I asked what her secret was, she reminded me that it's actually not her secret, but rather our mother-in-law's secret!

It's all about preparation.

And plastic bags.

But wait! Didn't I just get finished ranting about the evils of plastics in the last chapter? How can I justify using plastic bags?

My sister-in-law keeps fruits and veggies prechopped and neatly sealed in plastic bags; then when it's time to cook, all she has to do is pull out her "processed" (as in, processed by *her*) food and serve it or heat it up.

I watched her in action at our annual family summer get-together on the East Coast. Sure enough, "unzip" and *pow*, we've got salad. "Unzip" and *bam*, we've got fruit salad, too. In seconds.

Hmm, I thought to myself. *Maybe there's something to this plastic bag idea.*

But I was reluctant and resistant. Back home in my own mid-American kitchen, where I've done everything but hang a giant NO PLASTIC ALLOWED sign, I pondered the sister-in-law solution. That's when I got the idea to wrap my produce in waxed paper first, then put it in plastic. I would use plastic only when it wasn't a viable alternative to store something in a glass container, and then I would make sure there was always a layer of waxed paper between the food and the plastic. I also reuse the bags over and over until they are absolutely unusable.

The next part of my sister-in-law's equation was to never waste a chopping opportunity. For example, if I am preparing a salad for dinner, I always chop extra greens and veggies (not the ones that get soggy, like tomatoes); then I put everything I'm not using for the salad into my trusty glass containers or lined plastic bags. Voilà! Tomorrow's lunch or dinner is already half-finished. I can whip out an impressive spread just as effortlessly as my sister-in-law.

I've also started doing this with food for relish trays when I have parties. This keeps the stress level low for preparing for guests the day of an event.

I've utilized this concept for many special meals, and chopping, preparing, mixing, and making certain dishes ahead of time and refrigerating them has lightened my load significantly.

Now, I do realize that once you slice veggies, some of the nutrients are lost, but in my opinion, if slicing ahead of time reduces stress and encourages you to actually eat more salads, then the nutrient loss is a small price to pay. I've found there are days I don't mind cutting a fresh salad and then there are days when I would pay a million dollars (if I had a million dollars) for a live-in chef. Save your chopped veggies for *those* days. Just date your storage containers and use the oldest first.

Finally, I do have to say that if time is of the essence, there is absolutely nothing wrong with purchasing precut veggies and fruits at the store. You'll have the same minimal nutrient-loss issue and they'll cost a little more than buying the uncut veggies or fruits, but sometimes it's just worth it for the convenience. Rinse them and store in a glass container for use later. If you do buy precut veggies, it's best to use them within a day or two of purchase, just because they tend to get old quickly.

I Slaw It First!

I OFTEN MIX up a simple broccoli slaw salad for my husband that takes just minutes, because I use the packaged shredded broccoli slaw mix, and I add my own light homemade dressing of apple cider vinegar, olive oil, sea salt, agave nectar, and a dash of pepper. I whisk it all together and toss it with the bag of slaw. He eats the entire thing in one sitting—and it truly is faster than fast food. I'm done before I could have been to the drive-through and back again. My sons love it too, especially when I add some diced chicken and serve it for lunch. Expose your family to healthier foods that are quick for you to make, and you'll soon find out which are their new favorites.

THE BEAUTY OF SLOW FOOD

There is another side to the "Who has the time?" conundrum of preparing and eating whole foods. When it comes right down to it, my default method is almost always to just chop all the vegetables on a cutting board with my trusty old chef's knife. Even if it takes a long time. And here's why:

What you are doing is important.

You are preparing the food that will nourish you and your family. This is an *opportunity*. This is something you *get* to do. I know, I know, you're really busy, and *Dancing with the Stars* starts in forty-five minutes. But there are distinct and important (and beautifying! and slimming!) reasons to just *slow down*.

When you pay attention to what you are doing, you begin to interact with your food. You can appreciate the textures and colors, the sound of the knife, and the aromas that rise up out of a freshly cut vegetable.

I like to eat a ton of veggies in my salad, so it can take me a while to make one—I unwrap each vegetable, chop up the right amount, wrap the remaining vegetable up in waxed paper and then put it in a plastic bag, and then put it back in the refrigerator before I start on the next one. If you are the kind of person who makes a salad in a hurry, you probably wouldn't want to cook with me.

But to me, the process of chopping is almost like a meditation. It calms me and makes me feel relaxed. The rhythmic chopping, the bright colors and crisp textures, the simple beauty of the fresh vegetables and leafy greens, it's all part of the sensory experience.

If you really love to eat, then preparing the food can and should be part of that love.

And anyway, what's wrong with slowing down for one little part of your day? Your stress level will drop and your brain and body will thank you. And then you'll get to eat a really great salad. Isn't life nice? You might as well stop rushing through it and take a moment to smell the flowers . . . and the vegetables!

KEEPING WHOLE FOODS CLOSE AT HAND

All this talk about how much time it takes to prepare whole foods doesn't always apply, of course. Plenty of whole foods require no more than a quick rinse in the sink. Have them around all the time and they'll be the easiest thing for you and your kids to snack on. When it's quicker to grab a banana than run out to the store for a candy bar, I'm thinking you're going to go for the banana.

Other easy whole foods for your counter or the front of the refrigerator:

* Grapes
* Apples
* Pears
* Strawberries
* Blueberries
* Cubes or slices of melon
* Baby carrots
* Celery sticks
* Cucumber slices
* Cherry tomatoes
* Raisins
* Figs
* Dates

My grandmother used to peel and slice and serve me a bowl of cucumbers or apples every time we arrived for a visit, and those foods still evoke her presence for me. Watermelon and cantaloupe may be messy, but serving them on the rind makes preparation quicker and easier—and the fruit is just as delicious. These two are also great for preparing ahead of time and storing in glass containers.

To make whole-food snacks more appealing for you and the kids, involve them in the preparation. Even a two-year-old can help wash produce and tear lettuce leaves for salad. Being around food in this way can be fun and help root in children a healthy love of healthy food. (More on involving the little ones later in this chapter.)

GET FRESH!

Sometimes I get pretty fresh. Sometimes I'll even flirt shamelessly with my husband. The nerve of me! But right now, we're talking about whole foods, and another challenge you will probably encounter if you buy too many fruits and vegetables at the store.

They start to rot before you can eat them.

So let's talk about how to keep your produce not just ready to go but fresh as a daisy. Because nobody likes slimy cucumbers and dried-up baby carrots and fuzzy, blackish green . . . What *is* that stuff in that container? You don't even recognize it anymore.

According to the U.S. Environmental Protection Agency, Americans throw away nearly 31.6 million tons of food every year. That's a lot of food, Real Moms. A recent University of Arizona study found that the average family tosses 1.28 pounds of food a day, for a total of 470 pounds a year!

That's like throwing $600 directly into your garbage can.

I just know we can do something about this shameful waste. If we can figure out how to keep our food fresh until we eat it—all of it—then we won't be contributing to this massive problem.

So let's sit down, have a cup of green tea, and give this some serious thought. How many times have you suggested going out to dinner with your husband and kids while knowing good and well that you have chicken thawing in the refrigerator and lettuce practically begging to be eaten in the produce drawer? And then you go out to that restaurant and you order the chicken Caesar salad!

I can point the finger because I'm pointing it at myself! But be truthful. Why do this? Because 1) you didn't feel like cooking, and 2) you didn't feel like cleaning up after the meal, and 3) you wanted someone to just serve *you* for once, and 4) the restaurant's salads just taste better!

Fair enough. These are all perfectly valid reasons to want to go out to eat. But are they good enough reasons to actually do it?

Real Moms, listen up: We are in economically trying times. Save the money, spend the time, make people help you with the cleanup, and save the restaurant meals for when you *don't* have lettuce crying out for a salad bowl and a bit of dressing. If you begin to take pride in your cooking and you learn to make your salads taste even *better* than the ones in the restaurant, then you'll begin to feel cheated paying for something that isn't as good as you could get at home.

So set the table. Use the cloth napkins. Heck, why not light a candle? Decorate your precut lettuce with colorful chopped vegetables, pine nuts, a sprinkle of goat cheese. Warm your preroasted chicken breasts gently and sprinkle them with fresh herbs. Prepare a bit of pasta or a nice pilaf. And dine for a fraction of the cost! If you can get your husband to bring the food to the table and your kids to clear it off, then you've practically been waited on, and you won't even have to leave a tip (although hugs and kisses are always nice—and that waiter at the restaurant probably wouldn't even appreciate them!).

Here are a few more quick and easy solutions for keeping your whole foods fresh:

* I've found that if I wrap veggies, especially lettuce and celery, in a clean, dry paper towel and then place them back into the produce bag that has a few holes poked in it several inches apart, they stay fresher longer. Plus the paper towel acts as a barrier from the plastic (in lieu of the waxed paper). Consider using a paper towel that doesn't have bleaches or dye (coloring) to prevent the residue from getting on your produce. My friend swears by the same method, but she dampens the paper towel a bit to keep the freshness (moisture) locked into the bag. Each to his own! Whether to dampen the paper towel or not might depend on how humid your refrigerator is, and also on the weather.

* When you store produce in the refrigerator, remember to separate fruit and vegetables to different drawers, because the ethylene produced by the fruit will cause the vegetables to spoil more quickly.

* To store asparagus and herbs, snip off the ends and store them upright in a glass filled with about one inch of water. Cover with a plastic bag, or use an herb-saver container (like Prepara Herb-Savor Mini Pod—get it online at http://www.prepara.com/products/herb-savor-mini-pod/) made for this purpose. Replace the water daily.

* Don't cut into melons or squashes until you are ready to use them; then eat them up within a day or two.

* Did you know that direct sunlight keeps apples their freshest? Yep! Just arrange them in a pretty bowl on the countertop, near a sunny window, and let the sun work its natural magic. Pears, peaches, plums, and nectarines too.

Remember, in the olden days, there were no refrigerators, or they weren't that big (to store everything we do nowadays). Fruit grows outside in the sun. It likes the sun. Just don't buy more fruit than your family will eat in about a week.

* Always refrigerate berries, and keep them dry or they'll get moldy. Eat them within a couple of days. Cherries too. These are not long-lasting fruits.

THE EFFICIENCY EQUATION

Some Real Moms *love* to cook—but maybe not every single day of their lives for the next twenty years! Let's face it, sometimes even the most dedicated home cooks just want a break, but don't necessarily want to spring for a restaurant meal (or even put on shoes and find the car keys).

At the Institute for Integrative Nutrition, one of the recurring themes in our classes was the notion of cooking once, eating more than once. I discovered that before hearing this in class, I did it anyway, but hearing it out loud reinforced my healthy, eat-at-home, whole-food mentality even more. I realized that so many moms were slaving away in the kitchen when they should be out getting manicures (um . . . now?) or having family time or playing basketball and making mud pies with their kids (after which we will all need said manicure even more desperately).

The key to cooking once and eating twice goes beyond chopping extra vegetables whenever you happen to be chopping them, although that's a good start. Another trick is to spend one day making a few things that will last you all week.

For example, if you make a big pot of brown rice and roast a whole chicken on Sunday, you can probably get at least two and possibly three dinners out of that meal (unless you have teenage boys, in which case you'd better roast two chickens). Sunday dinner can be roast chicken with a fancy pilaf and a big salad. Monday might be chicken enchiladas with Spanish rice and refried beans.

On Tuesday, how about a big steaming pot of chicken-and-rice soup with veggies (precut ones, of course)?

Once you wrap your head around this concept, you'll be multi-mealing before you know it. We'll have an epidemic of moms with time on their hands! (So make your salon appointments quick.)

Brown rice is a great place to start practicing the multi-meal concept. Rice is a benign grain that most people like, and it's full of fiber and minerals. It's also got just over a hundred calories per half cup of cooked rice, and a nutty flavor you can grow to love, even if you think you're an instant-white-rice kind of mom.

Brown Rice Factoid

DID YOU KNOW that because of the oil in the bran layer of brown rice, it has a shorter shelf life than white rice? This means that it will maintain its quality for only about six months in the pantry. If you keep it in the freezer or refrigerator, you can store it up to a year.

Brown rice can stand in for white rice in any recipe; it tastes especially good in salads, stuffing, stews, and vegetarian dishes. Did you know that brown rice is available in three sizes? Yep, there's:

* **LONG-GRAIN:** Light, dry grains that separate easily when cooked. It's good under stir-fries or just in a bowl with a dab of butter and a sprinkle of herbs.
* **SHORT-GRAIN:** Fat, almost round grains with a higher starch content, which stick together when cooked and work well for sushi rolls.
* **MEDIUM-GRAIN:** Like baby bear's porridge, it's right between the other two extremes—"just right" for pilafs and for general use.

Rice is the perfect food to make while you are busy in the kitchen. Since it takes about forty-five minutes to cook, you have time to prepare the meat, cut the veggies (if you haven't already), and pull out the serving plates and storage containers for the next day's meal.

If you like rice and you make it often, consider springing for a rice cooker, which makes this job so easy and takes out all the trial and error. You can pick up a nice one at the department store—prices can range from $19.99 to upward of $100, depending on the bells and whistles, so, much like your juicer purchase, you can spend a little or a lot. Select one that fits your budget, or ask friends for the brands they like. Of course, a rice cooker is totally unnecessary. I don't have one and I make rice all the time, the old-fashioned way.

In that spirit, here is a basic recipe for preparing rice, in case you buy in bulk and store yours in glass containers like I do, and have long since discarded the plastic package with the preparation instructions:

BASIC BROWN RICE

■ **MAKES 3 TO 4 CUPS COOKED RICE, DEPENDING ON WHAT KIND OF RICE YOU USE.**

1 cup uncooked brown rice
2¼ cups liquid (water, broth)
1 tablespoon butter, margarine, or oil (optional)
1 teaspoon salt (optional)

Combine the rice, liquid, and optional fat and salt in a 2- to 3-quart saucepan. Heat to boiling; stir once or twice (stirring too much releases starch and makes the rice stickier), then reduce the heat to a simmer. Cover the pot and let it cook for about 45 minutes, or until the rice is tender and all the liquid is absorbed. Fluff with a fork and serve.

Store the brown rice you don't eat right away in a shallow container in the refrigerator for three to five days. According to the USA Rice Federation, cooked rice can also be stored in the freezer for six months. If you do choose to store in the freezer, cool the rice in the refrigerator first (get it in there within two hours), then transfer it to plastic freezer bags or freezable containers, in batches appropriate for individual meals. I like to label my rice with the date and quantity so I'll be ready to go without guessing when the need arises, *and* I can eat it within the six months.

Reheating rice for the next meal is simple. If you are making soup or any kind of cooked dish, you may not have to heat it on its own at all. Just use it straight out of the fridge. Or if you want to reheat it to eat it just the way it is, in all its simple riceness, just add two tablespoons of water per cup of rice, put it in a saucepan, and heat it up for about five minutes. Fluff with a fork, and add a little butter if you are feeling extra decadent. Enjoy!

Steamed Rice Is Also Nice

STEAMING IS A good way to warm up leftover rice, so if you love to use your steamer, try this easy dish: Cut up a zucchini, carrots, or any other firm fresh vegetable you happen to have on hand. Steam it along with a veggie burger for five minutes, then add a half cup of cooked rice to the steamer and steam for 2 more minutes. It's an almost-instant healthy meal! I like to top mine with a dash each of oil and vinegar and a sprinkle of pumpkin seeds, but you could garnish this dish in many ways. Thai-style peanut sauce? Mango chutney? Salsa? These are all premade, quick, and yummy.

MAKING THE MOST OF RICE

The first night that I make the rice, I usually serve it as, well . . . itself, in a pilaf as a basic side dish to my beef tenderloin and asparagus or roasted chicken and steamed broccoli and carrots, or whatever else I made for dinner. That's meal number one.

Then I get creative. Here are some of the recipes I've made with my leftover rice.

CINNAMON-RAISIN RICE PUDDING

■ SERVES 4.

2 cups cooked rice
2 cups milk (I like to use rice, soy, or almond milk)
¼ cup raisins
¼ cup maple syrup
1 tablespoon vanilla extract
1½ teaspoons cinnamon

Combine all the ingredients in a large saucepan. Bring to a boil over medium-high heat, stirring constantly, then reduce heat to low and simmer for 15 minutes, or until the pudding has a nice, creamy, thickened consistency. Delicious hot or cold, for breakfast, lunch, dinner, or a midnight snack.

Here's another leftover rice recipe I love, adapted from one published by the USA Rice Foundation. The almonds and sunflower seeds give it texture, crunch, flavor, and extra nutrients.

HEALTH NUT BROWN RICE

■ SERVES 6.

1 tablespoon olive oil
⅓ cup sliced almonds
⅓ cup sunflower kernels
⅓ cup julienned carrots (cut them into long thin strips, like matchsticks)
¼ teaspoon red pepper flakes (optional)
3 cups cooked brown rice
2 tablespoons chopped fresh parsley

1. Heat the olive oil in a large skillet over medium-high heat. Add the almonds and sunflower kernels. Stir until the almonds and sun-

flower seeds start to turn golden-brown, but watch them carefully so they don't burn—this should take only a couple of minutes.

2. Add the carrots and optional red pepper flakes. Stir to coat. Add the brown rice and stir to combine everything. Heat until the rice is completely cooked through.

3. Stir in the fresh parsley and serve warm.

Stir-fry, No Recipe Required

SOMETIMES USING LEFTOVER rice doesn't even require a recipe. Just stir-fry diced chicken, soy sauce, and a pinch of powdered ginger with chopped vegetables like broccoli, carrots, onions, green beans, and asparagus. Serve over reheated rice. Easy-peasy, and so delicious.

I hope this has inspired you to cook once and eat two, three, four times or more. You could do the same thing with a big batch of any grain, like quinoa, bulgur wheat, millet, or polenta. It would also work with couscous or even stubby pasta. When you use one food element as the basis for several meals, life gets easier and you end up eating fresh, whole, healthy foods more often.

And you thought it was going to be hard.

CALL IN THE REINFORCEMENTS!

My children are a little bit older now, but when they were toddlers, I purchased them a set of wooden "produce" toys, with Velcro in between the fabricated "cuts." With a little wooden knife, they would cut and cut to their heart's desire, "helping" me make dinner while I chopped the real vegetables with the real knife. They would watch, fascinated, as I cut vegetables for salads or fruit for the dinner table, and all three of them now know exactly what happens before mealtime—you chop, and then you cook.

This training has made them willing helpers in the kitchen, and I strongly encourage all Real Moms to get their kids into the kitchen and lending little helping hands as early as possible. Depending on how old your kids are, they can do many different kitchen jobs, if you just set up a space for them.

When my boys were a bit older and wanted to help with the real food, I would give them a carrot, a veggie brush, and a big bowl of water, and they would scrub away. (Scrubbing carrots leaves more nutrients behind than peeling, and besides, those vegetable peelers are sharp!)

At the next stage of maturity, I let them use spoons to scoop the seeds from cantaloupes and watermelons. Then I let them use butter knives to spread jam or peanut butter on bread. They could pour the water into the glasses (not the lemonade, those spills are stickier!), and they always enjoyed mixing up a batch of trail mix for snacks. I'd provide the bags, jars, and boxes of granola, raisins, dried cranberries, almonds, walnuts, and chocolate or carob chips, and let them do the mixing with a big bowl and a wooden spoon. They got to decide on the ratios, so the trail mix became the result of their own invented "recipe."

These days, my kids are pretty mature and can handle most cooking chores. Today, my oldest son cuts my youngest son's pancakes into bite-size pieces, and my middle son sets the table. I let them contribute to the creation of our family meal plans, so they are part of the process from the very beginning. After all, they're eating the food too. They should have a say in what we make, and I want them to enjoy it as much as I do. (Real Kids love to eat too!)

My oldest son is a whiz at math, and when I have a kitchen calculation, he's my go-to guy for figuring it out (what's two-thirds of a cup times four?). The youngest is very creative, so when I want an extraspecial table setting, he's the man for the job (nice homemade place mats!). I love it when one of my sons will go to the grocery store with me. "Dividing and conquering" is better than spending an hour in the grocery store—there's so much more fun to be had making and eating the food. My sons have learned to pick out perfectly ripe produce while I select the meats and fish.

Every once in a while I tell the boys it's backward day (usually when Dad's not around) and we go out for ice cream or some other luscious dessert and then eat dinner (or something substantial) later.

Because dinner can't be *all* about vegetables.

BUT MY KIDS DON'T *WAAAAAANT* TO HELP!

It's not that my kids are so perfect. Most kids will try to get out of unpleasant work, so the trick to getting the help you need in the kitchen is to make it pleasant. Here are some tips:

* **BE SPECIFIC:** Children like concise, clear directives. Instead of, "Clean the kitchen!" which is so general (I don't like that directive either!), be more specific. For instance, say, "Please carry the plates to the sink, rinse them off with the dish brush, and put them in the dishwasher," or, "Please put all the condiments back into the refrigerator." This will eliminate your frustration when they don't do things the way you like them to be done, it will give them a feeling of accomplishment, and it gets the jobs done very quickly. I've even thought about typing out and laminating the steps to preparing, cooking, and cleaning the kitchen, so my sons will remember what to do—but I'm still thinking about the best way to do that. Maybe you've got an idea?

* **CREATIVITY ROCKS:** Kids love to play and be creative, so bring that spirit into the kitchen. I learned this when I sent my youngest child to a cooking camp and spied on the teachers—they let the kids create their own meals in the most nontraditional and creative ways, without ever telling anybody they were doing anything wrong. My son *still* talks about how much he loved that experience. When I give my kids an assigned kitchen task, I really try to back off (I lock the controlling part of myself up in my room for a "time-out"), stop micromanaging or criticizing, and let them do what comes naturally to them. So they don't tear up the lettuce the way you would? They don't set the table correctly and everyone has to quietly move their forks to the *other* side of the plate? So they make a bit of a mess? So what?! Creativity makes everything more fun.

* **TEENS CAN LEARN TOO:** Teenagers don't always want to get involved, so it's best to instill these behaviors at a young

age, when they can learn to enjoy it. But you can still enlist your teens, prefaced by the whole "you're old enough to help out more around the house now" lecture. Just remember to let them be creative too.

* **TAKE REQUESTS:** I make it a personal rule that when my sons request a certain meal, I try to make it. I know that when I have a craving for a certain food, it's hard to deny it, and so I imagine that if they took the time to come out and ask for it, it must be something they really want or need. (Candy and ice cream don't count—but I do allow those every so often, on special occasions!)

* **SAFETY FIRST:** I try not to control the situation too much in the kitchen, but rather stand by as a silent observer (sometimes forcibly zipping my lip!). I do, however, require standard food safety and health rules, such as hand washing. I've hounded them so many times that the moment they enter the house, they go straight to the sink to wash up (soap, water, and completely dry)—good for them!

My sons sure learned about safety in the kitchen one day when I was making something hot in a fry pan and the handle was not pushed toward the middle of the stove; I walked by and caught the handle with the sleeve of my "big" sweater and nearly dropped the pan and its contents to the floor. Luckily, I caught the pan before it fell, but the entire house heard me shriek, and the results could have been much more disastrous.

Another time, my youngest son (as a toddler) was pulling himself to a standing position around my ankles in the kitchen while I was loading the dishwasher. In an instant, his feet slipped out from under him and he pitched face-first into the silverware basket of the dishwasher. The neighbors probably heard that scream, followed by my loud pronouncement: "And *that's* why Mommy always puts the knives *pointdown* in the silverware basket!" Still, it almost gave me a heart attack. His little face had a tiny red mark from the handle of the knife, but again, this could have been a much more tragic story.

* **EMBRACE *MISE EN PLACE*:** When the kids want to help with a

recipe, I bring out my cooking school concept, *mise en place*—a French phrase defined by the Culinary Institute of America as "everything in place." This means getting all the ingredients for a recipe set out and measured before starting to cook. Kids are great at preparing the *mise en place*. Then, when I (or we) start cooking, everything goes smoothly.

I remember one time, I was making a quick batch of chocolate-chip cookies for my sons before I left to pick them up at school. I'd already cracked open the eggs when I realized I had no brown sugar. If I had prepared my *mise en place* before I started cooking, I wouldn't have been stuck mid-recipe with no brown sugar. I had to run to the store, buy brown sugar, pick up the kids, and guess what? They made the cookies for me! (Hey, maybe that wasn't such a bad plan after all. . . .)

* **ATTEMPT TO KEEP IT CLEAN:** I've long given up on the concept that my sons will wear an apron, but if your kids do, great! Instead, I usually end up washing chocolate or tomato sauce out of their T-shirts.

* **INSTITUTE A POLICY: NO ONE'S FINISHED UNTIL WE'RE ALL FIN-ISHED!:** That's my policy in the kitchen. My children are all old enough now to know that they don't leave a mess behind for me to clean up alone. I'll pay you a hundred bucks if one of my sons doesn't help you clean up in the kitchen. I'm not bragging; I'm just illustrating that if you teach your kids to help clean up when they are young, they will just assume it's something that must be done, like brushing their teeth or changing their underwear.

By working together, food prep, mealtime, and cleanup can be a snap, leaving more time for family game night!

DO FIVE THINGS

You're ready. I just know it. Ready to make 80 percent of your diet whole food. You can *do this*! But you can do it gradually too. Here are five ways to make it happen this week:

1. EXPAND YOUR PRODUCE REPERTOIRE. FIND A NEW FRUIT OR VEGETABLE YOU'VE NEVER TRIED, LEARN HOW TO PREPARE IT, AND GIVE IT A TRY.

Whether it's pomegranates or parsnips or something completely different, get a little daring this week. Google your produce of choice and find some cool things to do with it.

2. PRECUT VEGETABLES FOR SALADS OR SNACKS AT THE BEGINNING OF THE WEEK, AND KEEP THEM FRESH WITH THIS TRICK.

Thirty minutes of chopping on a Sunday will keep your family in fresh, healthy, whole-food snacks all week long.

3. COOK ONCE; EAT TWO OR EVEN THREE TIMES.

Follow the directions in this chapter for making a big batch of rice or other grains, then use it for several meals. Roast a chicken or even a turkey or a big salmon fillet. And don't forget all those prechopped veggies. Dinner in a snap, and you'll save money too.

4. BRING IN THE REINFORCEMENTS! WHY SHOULD YOU HAVE TO DO IT ALL ALONE?

Your kids want to spend time with you. What better place than in the kitchen?

5. I KNOW YOU ARE STILL DRINKING YOUR EIGHT GLASSES OF FRESH, PURE WATER EVERY DAY. IS IT A HABIT YET?

Keep going with this—it will make every part of your body work better!

WEEK NINE:

Go Out on the Town

THIS WEEK, DO FIVE THINGS:

1. Before you go out, look at the restaurant's menu ahead of time on the Internet, or call ahead to ask whether the chef is amenable to special orders. This will help avoid a scene when you try to order, steer you away from the places that aren't for you, and banish forever the notion that you can't eat healthy *and* eat out.

2. Order large or go home! Always order enough to take half of your meal home for lunch the next day. Two meals for the price of one.

3. Try a new entrée that you've never eaten before. Be adventurous! You are ready.

4. When in Rome . . . If you are invited to someone's home for dinner, or invited out to dinner, roll with the punches. Remember, it's what you do 80 percent of the time that counts. Just eat what you want to eat. Enjoy yourself! You deserve it.

5. Isn't it great that you're still drinking your eight glasses of fresh, pure water every day?

OH, THE THRILL of love! You know how it is. You can't get enough of your beloved—all you want to do is hunker down at home and relish the deliciousness, each moment a precious, unforgettable eternity. You're so smitten and single-minded, you forget all about the outside world.

But at some point, you're going to want to go out again.

I just know that you're as madly in love with whole food as I am, by this point. And what great confidence you've gained as you practice your new cooking skills! But . . . is it confession time again? As you've probably surmised from my oblique (or not so oblique) references to the wonders and joys of being served by waiters in a restaurant . . .

I love to go out to eat!

I admit it! Yes, I do! The hosts! The lovely dining rooms! The wine! The waiters! The service! The busboys! The fact that *they clean it all up for you afterward*! Alas, it's true. I'm smitten with eating out. It may not be the most cost-effective way to eat, and don't get me wrong; I'm all about my home-cooked whole foods, but while whole food is my dietary life partner, going out to eat is my celebrity crush.

I don't do it every day. But every so often? I maintain that Real Moms don't just want but *require* a little bit of good service every now and again. It's worth every penny of that 20 percent tip.

However, eating out can also become a dietary land mine, if you aren't careful. Restaurant food can be astonishingly high in fat, salt, and sugar. Why do you think it tastes so good? Also, when you aren't making the food yourself, you don't know what exactly is in that cassoulet or pasta dish or even what was used to grill that lovely salmon fillet. Was it olive oil? Butter? Cheap vegetable oil? How much salt is in that dish? How much sugar? What kind of spices, flavorings, colorings? Where did they get their ingredients?

But never fear. You *can* go out to eat at restaurants and still maintain your healthy whole-foods lifestyle.

Always eat a little bit lighter on the days you know you will be dining at a restaurant. When you'll be having lunch out, have a light breakfast, but don't *skip* breakfast. Make sure you have some protein and fiber, so you aren't famished and tempted to overorder and stuff yourself. A smoothie with protein powder is perfect.

If you'll be eating out for dinner, have a lighter lunch. An apple with nut butter, a half cup of yogurt or cottage cheese and some applesauce, or whole-grain crackers with hummus are all good choices. Then you can have fun going out to eat and focus on your husband or your friends without obsessing over the fine print on the menu and then ordering two of everything.

Once you get to the restaurant, you'll have the greatest success if you feel confident enough to order well. And by well, I mean *annoyingly*.

CHANNELING MEG RYAN

Remember that scene in the classic movie *When Harry Met Sally* when Meg Ryan—no, not *that* scene, where she pretends to have an, um . . . erotic experience in the diner. I mean the one where she orders from the restaurant menu and picks apart every aspect of the dish she wants, asking for all kinds of changes and special considerations?

That's me! If I tally up the number of times I've annoyed and probably completely embarrassed my husband on our date night by special-ordering at the restaurant, I could count them on both hands, and my husband's hands, and the hands of all three of my kids. And then some.

Real Moms should get what they want!

I'm not saying you should be rude. Not at all! In fact, picky restaurant eaters are, in my opinion, obliged to be *extra* polite, and fully cognizant that they may be slightly more high-maintenance than other diners, that this takes the waiter's time, and that you appreciate this deeply.

But you should still get what you want.

This is me:

"I'll have the chicken, but without mushrooms, onions on the side, olive oil instead of butter, no butter in the dish at all, please, and can you tell the chef to salt it lightly? And as for the salad, please leave out the croutons, and could I have extra tomatoes? Oh, and can you check whether your salad dressing contains high-fructose corn syrup? Because if it does, I'd prefer just a little olive oil and red wine vinegar on the side, please. And thank you *so much* for putting up with these requests; I really appreciate it a great deal!" (Follow with radiant smile.)

Being choosy in a restaurant isn't about dieting. It's about your well-being and personal satisfaction. Eating out is expensive under the best of circumstances, compared with eating at home, so why do it if you aren't going to get food you love, prepared the way you like it (even if it means your dining companions are rolling their eyes and emitting deep existential sighs)?

Because, you see, I don't like mushrooms. I like my onions doled out sparingly. I prefer the taste and health benefits of olive oil to butter, I don't want to be bloated from too much salt, I don't like croutons enough to make them worth the starch, I love tomatoes, and I prefer to keep my system free of high-fructose corn syrup.

Is that so wrong?

If you pay a premium for a good restaurant meal, you should get the food you want, the way you want it, with no surprises.

RESTAURANT WISDOM

You might not be as picky as I am, or maybe you are even choosier about exactly how your food is prepared. Either way, you can get more out of your restaurant experience, and less bloating and fewer bad feelings the next day, by following a few simple Real Moms Love to Eat guidelines.

1. READ THE MENU ONLINE. I almost always do this before I go out to eat, because I want to be able to plan what I will order ahead of time, and give it some thought. Then I can be prepared when I get to the restaurant, and I won't take quite so long to order (I like to read the *whole* menu before I choose!). My husband appreciates this small consideration, especially since he already knows he's going to have to endure my giving the waiter the third degree (he has perfected his silent sympathetic look on behalf of waitstaff everywhere).

If I don't see something I want, sometimes I'll call the restaurant and ask if it would be possible to get what I *do* want. If they give me a hard time, I am tipped off that the service might not be so great, and maybe we'll go somewhere else. If they are polite and accommodating, then in my mind, the tip has already gone up.

2. ASK QUESTIONS. When I get to the restaurant, I always ask a lot of questions. Why shouldn't I? I want to know what's in the dishes, and sometimes I want to know if my special requests can be accommodated. If I've had a carb-heavy day, will they leave the bread basket off the table? Are they willing to go lighter on oil or salt? Could they leave off the potatoes and give me double the green beans? It never hurts to ask, as long as you ask nicely.

If you have dietary preferences, or, in the cases of allergies and intolerances, dietary *requirements*, then you have the right to have those needs met. If you want your meal to be vegetarian, ask for this. If you need dairy-free or gluten-free, ask! If you want to feel light and good and not heavy and weighed down, then you have the right to ask for your food to be prepared with less fat, salt, and sugar. Ask about ingredients, how the food is cooked, and whether there are any "secret" ingredients that aren't listed on the menu.

Recently, I looked up a restaurant's menu online before I went there for lunch, so I knew exactly what I was going to order: the Caesar salad. When it arrived at the table, however, I was surprised to see black olives, roasted red peppers, and capers all over it.

Some days I might have eaten it, but I was not in an adventurous mood, and the menu had said nothing about the inclusion of these rogue Mediterranean ingredients! Not that there is anything wrong with olives and roasted red peppers, but it wasn't what I wanted, and I also felt duped. The menu should disclose the ingredients in a dish! I wanted just a simple Caesar salad with chicken. (No croutons. Dressing on the side.)

I sent it back, but I also learned my lesson: If you don't like surprises, and especially if you aren't a particularly adventurous eater, always ask whether there is anything on the salad that the menu doesn't list. Better safe than stuck with a salad covered in something icky.

Send It Back . . . with a Caveat!

I HAVE A friend who is so sure that if she gives the waiter or waitress any trouble, they will spit in her food when they bring it back. Because of this fear, she'll accept and eat food even if it isn't what she wanted or she doesn't like it.

I say, don't let a restaurant bully you! If you're going to go out to eat, don't go to the spots where you doubt the integrity of the staff or the hygienic practices in the kitchen. Go to a good restaurant with good food and a sterling reputation, and then enjoy yourself. Sometimes you really do get what you pay for.

3. EAT FOR ONE. Most restaurant meals give you enough food to feed your whole family, but since it's tacky to order one entrée for you, your husband, and all your children, a better way to keep from overstuffing yourself is to take home half your meal, every time.

I make this an almost sacred rule. Consider it a riff on the cook-once-eat-twice idea from chapter eight. Even if I think I could eat the whole meal, I know that half of that same meal will feel like plenty of food when I get to the end of it. This is an easy way to cut back without missing anything.

And, in fact, you're gaining something delicious! I am a big fan of restaurant leftovers. I love the taste of salmon or chicken the next day, even cold, out of the refrigerator. It's lunch without effort, and you're getting two meals for the price of one. Genius!

4. APPETIZERS ARE APPETIZING. The average size of a hamburger in the 1950s was just 1.5 ounces. Today they can weigh in at eight ounces or even more—I've seen ⅔-pound burgers on more than a few restaurant menus. Yikes! If you know you won't be able to eat those leftovers the next day for whatever reason, consider ordering from the appetizer menu. Nobody said you have to order an entrée. Not only are the appetizers generally much less expensive, but you'll probably get plenty of food. Unless you really, really want them, avoid the deep-fat-fried appetizers (like the basket of fries, onion rings, poppers, and fried mushrooms), just because those are way overloaded with fat and salt. Instead, look for yummy lean, fresh appetizers like chicken on skewers with peanut sauce, roasted beets with goat cheese, flatbread topped with shrimp or crab and a little cheese, sweet potato fries (preferably baked), or, of course, the old standbys, soup and salad. I also like tapas-style restaurants, where you can order several small plates of delicious fresh food, Spanish-style. More and more restaurants are accommodating people with smaller appetites and varied tastes these days. What a great trend!

5. DON'T BE SHY. After all my talk of being a picky eater, I do believe it's also great to have a sense of adventure when you are eating out. One of the best things about restaurants is that you have the opportunity to be exposed to foods you might never have thought to try, or wouldn't have the first idea how to cook.

I have been lucky enough to "work" as a secret restaurant rater for a certain Chicago restaurant conglomerate. That means I get to go out to eat and submit a review, rating the service, food, and entire restaurant experience—and then I get reimbursed for the expense! It's a dream job for a Real Mom who loves to eat, but one of the things I love the most about it is that I am "required" to try new foods I would not ordinarily eat. I am obligated to order and eat an appetizer, entrée, wine (if applicable), and dessert. Poor me!

For my report, I have to assess flavor, texture, ambience, service, and everything else that would be relevant to others wanting to know whether they should visit a particular restaurant. First, I look at the plate as it's brought to the table, and assess the presentation. Next, I take a bite. I try to detect the flavors. Sometimes I ask the server questions, like, "Do I detect a hint of cinnamon? Cayenne? Cumin?" (Yes, my husband is rolling his eyes again!) I determine how well the dish pairs with the suggested wine. I analyze the dessert.

But you don't have to be a restaurant rater to bring this same level of attention, analysis, and sensual enjoyment to your own restaurant meal. Be daring; try something new. Duck? Mussels? Quinoa? Go ahead; order the appetizer, the entrée, the wine, *and* the dessert. You have my full support, as a fellow Real Mom! It might be an indulgence, but it won't be an overindulgence, especially if you are saving half for tomorrow, and not going out for dinner every night. The occasional special meal is a wonderful part of life, and nobody should have to miss out on the special moments.

6. CELEBRATE THE CUISINE. Why go to a seafood restaurant for a hamburger, or an Italian restaurant for rice? I love to order what the restaurant does best, while also keeping healthful eating at the top of my list.

I am obsessed with all things French, and every so often, I indulge in a beautiful dinner at a French bistro. To eat well at a French restaurant, do as the French do: Eat tiny portions! They are so sweet and stylish, with their tiny bits of gorgeous food on beautiful plates. Shouldn't Real Moms *always* eat this way? *Oui!* I usually have only a tiny bit of the rich cream sauces and focus on the elegant vegetable creations.

At a Chinese restaurant, I often ask them to hold the rice or noodles. I order the mixed vegetables with nuts or a chicken entrée (not the deep-fat-fried kind) with a wine-based sauce, rather than one of the sweeter sauces. I'll share the huge portion with my husband (or bring half home). I always try to eat with chopsticks too. It makes me feel like I'm getting a more authentic experience, and it also slows me down. One of my favorite things to order in a Chinese restaurant is wonton soup and cucumber salad or lettuce wraps.

Say "pasta with red sauce" and I'm yours. I remember when I was training for the Boston Marathon, I'd get my husband to take me out for Italian every night for days. While Americans tend to envision Italian food as giant plates of pasta, the truth is that in Italy, lean protein usually takes center stage, and pasta is a side dish, along with plenty of fresh, delicious vegetables. Two of my favorite Italian dishes are Mozzarella alla Caprese and Chicken Parmesan. For years, my husband and I have frequented Maggiano's Little Italy in Chicago. Their Chicken Parmesan is heavenly— it's breaded and sautéed, topped with melted cheese and a bold marinara sauce . . . not a particularly low-calorie or low-fat choice, but definitely worth the occasional indulgence . . . *delizioso!*

I'm a big fan of Mexican food, and I almost always order a delicious margarita with high-end tequila (I'm a lightweight; I can usually handle only one!). Freshly fried tortilla chips and a little salsa, and I'm doing a hat dance before you can say *olé*! I love the spices and heat of Mexican food, and I usually focus my meals on the black-bean salsas and chicken or beef fajitas, hold the tortillas. I ask for extra onions and peppers and skip the rice too, or ask for lettuce to make lettuce wraps. I find that if I avoid the starchy dishes, I feel much better the next morning.

American-style bistros generally do a great job with soup. One of my favorite types is butternut squash, and I think Chicago-based Charlie Trotter's does it best! Or I'll get a broth-based soup rather than a cream soup, just because I find it equally yummy but with a lot less fat and fewer calories. Might as well cut back when it doesn't influence my enjoyment of the meal! I also love chili.

I don't eat Indian food that often, but I have plenty of friends who adore it. One of my girlfriends dines out at Indian restaurants at least twice a week. Sometimes she gets the fried dishes, but often she enjoys dishes centered around vegetables and legumes, some with no meat at all. Many of the curries and roasted meat dishes are full of vegetables and lean protein, and some are entirely vegetarian and superlight but highly flavorful. With fragrant basmati rice and a bit of soft warm naan bread on the side, it's the perfect cuisine for vegetarians and people who like it spicy.

And when you're stuck at the mall or the food court in the airport? It's still possible to have a relatively healthy meal. Hunt for a baked potato, a small hamburger, a deli sandwich on whole-grain bread (hold the creamy sauces and add more veggies), a veggie pizza, bean burrito, barbecued or grilled chicken sandwich, salad (hold the croutons and creamy dressing), or a cup of frozen yogurt. If I know I'm going to the mall, sometimes I'll just eat ahead of time, or stick a healthy snack bar or a zippered bag full of homemade trail mix in my purse.

THWARTING THE BUFFET BOOBY TRAP

My family *loves* to take me out for a big Mother's Day brunch at a swanky buffet. I know they have good intentions, but this is always a tough one for me. I want to feel good on Mother's Day, not stuffed to the gills, even if it's with the best food. Do I really need seven plates of food? For one meal? Does *anyone*?

You may face a similar situation whenever your family goes out for a special occasion to any all-you-can-eat kind of restaurant. Something about holidays and celebrations flips a switch in our brains and we tend to think it's okay to eat huge amounts of food. It's the *Supersize Me* mentality. There is nothing wrong with celebrating, but can you have your cake and eat it and not eat the *whole cake*?

Of course you can! You can even go back up to the buffet *three times*, and still leave feeling great. Here's how to visit a buffet, have a great time, and still eat like a lady. Because the fancy shoes and the Easter dress do not constitute a license to gorge.

Trip Number One: Hooray, the buffet! After the initial excitement, the holiday chatter, and getting seated, take a few deep calming breaths so you have your wits about you, then head straight to the salad bar. Starting with a salad will fill you up with healthy vegetables before you even *look* at the dessert table. Load up on fresh greens and fresh veggies. Avoid the mayo-laden salads and creamy dressings. Go for carrots, radishes, bell peppers, beets, broccoli, cauliflower, and maybe a few sunflower seeds, raisins, or olives, if you like them. Drizzle with vinaigrette. In your *other hand* (you're two-fisting it already, you party animal, you!), get a cup of brothy soup, like chicken noodle, vegetable beef, or Manhattan clam chowder. Meander back to the table. Eat it all! Oh, Real Moms, you are *virtue incarnate*.

Trip Number Two: Time to head to the carving station! Get a nice palm-size piece of thinly sliced roast beef, turkey, or ham. Now, what kind of delicious steamed or grilled vegetables might go with that? Green beans? Broccoli and carrots? Cauliflower? If you really want it, add a small spoonful of rice or mashed potatoes, or even bread stuffing, but make sure most of what's on your plate is those veggies. Go back to the table and savor every bite, but don't feel like you have to finish everything on your plate. Stop when you've had enough.

Trip Number Three: Do you still have room for dessert? Think about whether you really want it. If you don't, order a cup of tea or coffee and treat it like dessert. If you do, then go for it! Use a small dessert plate and pick the one or two things that you really, really want. (I would tell you to just go for the mixed berries, but I have a feeling you'd throw your dinner roll at me!) It's a holiday, and you *do* deserve a treat, so go ahead! Just don't finish it if you really don't want every single bite. Pay attention to how you are feeling. Eating is fun, but feeling stuffed isn't.

There, now, wasn't that fun? You indulged, you made multiple trips to the buffet, and everybody feels like they really got to celebrate. You weren't sitting at the table picking at your single plate of meager fixings and making everybody else feel like you are deprived. You enjoyed yourself, and that helped everybody else have more fun too. Happy Mother's Day! (Or whatever the occasion is.)

OPP (OTHER PEOPLE'S PARTIES)

Restaurants are fine and good for being picky. After all, you're paying the bill. But what happens when you go to someone else's home for a dinner party, or you attend an event like a wedding, where everyone is being served the same food, or you're faced with (gasp!) *the dreaded buffet*, full of dietary catastrophes with potentially thousands of calories per nibble?

Don't panic! I've got your back.

You can't exactly send your wedding reception plate of food back, demanding a special order. That would just be rude. And although not everyone agrees with me, I don't think you should ever demand special concessions from your host at a dinner party. Real Moms live in the real world, and being a guest in someone's home or at someone else's celebration is an honor and a privilege. It's not a time to be demanding all the attention because you can't eat this or won't eat that.

Before I really learned how to embrace the Real Moms Love to Eat way of life, I used to visit family and be so darned difficult that I'd bring my own stash of food that I just knew would be healthier and lower in fat and calories than what I would be served. My mom probably used to shudder when I would visit her in her beautiful home in Phoenix. As soon as I walked in the door, I would announce that I was going shopping for "healthy food." What a pain in the ass I was! Sheesh. Now *I'm* rolling my eyes at myself!

I've lightened up, figuratively *and* literally, as I've learned that as long as I am eating clean whole foods 80 percent of the time, the rest of the time I can just relax and go with the flow. Think about it—nine times out of ten, you probably break your own eating rules anyway, so why suddenly get so puritanical in front of others? *Obnoxious!*

Thank goodness for family forgiveness and the love and understanding of mothers, or I'd probably be ousted from the family by now. Today, when I visit my mother, I'll eat her awesome homemade cookies, chocolate-covered raisins, roasted turkey, and whatever else she made. No more subjecting others to my picky eating. Sorry, Mom!

Family and friends shouldn't have to worry about what you are eating. If you or your child has a food allergy, of course, that's a different story, but if you are just trying to lose weight or be healthier, it's definitely not worth insulting or even inconveniencing your gracious host.

Instead, just eat moderately. It's that simple. Have a little of everything, and politely decline seconds because you are just so full from the absolutely delicious food that you couldn't possibly eat another bite.

'Nuff said.

DO FIVE THINGS

Are you already on the phone making restaurant reservations? Good for you! Because this week, you are *assigned* to eat out. Just remember to do these five things:

1. BEFORE YOU GO OUT, LOOK AT THE RESTAURANT'S MENU AHEAD OF TIME ON THE INTERNET, OR CALL AHEAD TO ASK WHETHER THE CHEF IS AMENABLE TO SPECIAL ORDERS.

This will help avoid a scene when you try to order, steer you away from the places that aren't for you, and banish forever the notion that you can't eat healthy and eat out. Plan what you will order ahead of time, but also be flexible. Sometimes online menus aren't updated, and the restaurant menu may not be exactly the same. Pick out several things you might like and decide ahead of time about any special requests you might have. Then, when you get to the restaurant, smile, be nice, be polite, be compassionate to the waiter and complimentary to the chef when warranted, and you'll have a great time! Everyone at your table will be grateful.

2. ORDER LARGE OR GO HOME! ALWAYS ORDER ENOUGH TO TAKE HALF OF YOUR MEAL HOME FOR LUNCH THE NEXT DAY. TWO MEALS FOR THE PRICE OF ONE.

This week, when you eat out, ask for a to-go box when you order. Put half your meal into it and set it aside before you begin eating. And don't forget to bring it with you at the end of the meal! (I can't tell you how many to-go boxes I've left on the restaurant table, only to remember them the next day when I was eager for my lunch of restaurant leftovers. Darn it!)

3. TRY A NEW ENTRÉE THAT YOU'VE NEVER EATEN BEFORE. BE ADVENTUROUS! YOU ARE READY.

You *are* ready. Go for the skate, the guinea hen, the portabella burger, the amaranth pilaf. You might find a new favorite, and even if you don't, you'll feel proud of yourself. (A friend of mine recently ordered sweetbreads, thinking they were a dessert. Boy, was she surprised to find out she ate calf pancreas! But now she brags about it.)

4. WHEN IN ROME . . . IF YOU ARE INVITED TO SOMEONE'S HOME FOR DINNER, OR INVITED OUT TO DINNER, ROLL WITH THE PUNCHES. REMEMBER, IT'S WHAT YOU DO 80 PERCENT OF THE TIME THAT COUNTS. JUST EAT WHAT YOU WANT TO EAT. ENJOY YOURSELF! YOU DESERVE IT.

And so does your gracious host or hostess. (Don't forget the hostess gift!)

5. ISN'T IT GREAT THAT YOU'RE STILL DRINKING YOUR EIGHT GLASSES OF FRESH, PURE WATER EVERY DAY?

Sometimes I wonder what my life would be like if I hadn't formed and maintained my water habit with so much diligence. It's such an important part of my day. During the afternoon, I drink it with slices of cucumber or grapefruit or a sliced strawberry—a virginal sort of cocktail. I also recently installed a filter, so I can drink the tap water and know it's pure.

Hey, this week was *fun*, and you got to go out to eat just for the sake of practicing your new Real Moms Love to Eat lifestyle. I hope you're realizing how easy it is to take this "diet" on the road. Anywhere you go, you can indulge in mostly fresh, real food, enjoy your meals without guilt, and feel great. You can go to parties, weddings, formal dinners, and any kind of restaurant on the planet, because you know how to make smart choices and order well. Go ahead. You're not afraid. You eat danger for *dinner*. (With a side of steamed vegetables, please. No butter.)

WEEK TEN:

Explore the Ethics of Eating

> THIS WEEK, DO FIVE THINGS:
>
> 1. Go to your local farmers' market and purchase at least one locally produced vegetable or fruit. Talk to the farmer and get to know the source of your food.
> 2. Switch at least three foods in your pantry/refrigerator to organic. I'll tell you which choices will make the most difference to your health *and* the planet.
> 3. Look at the packaging on your food. Is it earth-friendly? I'll show you how to tell.
> 4. Go veg once a week . . . then twice.
> 5. Thank goodness you're still drinking your eight glasses of fresh, pure water every day!

A T SOME POINT, every woman involved in a torrid affair is bound to question the ethics of her involvement. Is all this pleasure . . . *allowed*? Even more important, are you living your beliefs when you eat your meals?

I'm the first one to stand up and say, "Yes! Pleasure is *allowed*!" But I also have strong feelings about certain issues that impact my food choices, and those help to keep me from jumping into the pleasure deep end. For me, the most important thing a Real Mom can do is to work to keep food and the environment pure, clean, healthy, and kind, for the sake of the next generation. Because let's face it, Real Moms—we're talking about our kids. If our generation trashes the planet, where are our children, and their children, and their children, going to live? How will they get to grow up happy, healthy, and appreciative of all that the planet has to give us if we've tapped it all out? (They don't call me the Green Mom for nothing!)

That's my big platform, but each Real Mom will have those food-related issues that resonate with her. Is it pesticides? Food waste? The cruelty of and/or the pollution from factory farms and feedlots? Is it child health? Poverty? People in your own community who don't have enough to eat? Is it artificial or chemically derived ingredients, or the importance of local or organic foods?

Think about what you really believe in, and whether you are doing anything about it, because Real Moms who act on what they believe not only make the world better, but set a good example for their children by sending the message that you *can* change things.

Because you *can*.

Fortunately, you can also maintain your fondness for pleasure at the table. You can do right by your family, your community, and your planet and also love food, eat food, and revel in the delicious nature of food. This chapter will get you thinking about the big picture of eating, from the cleanliness of the bite on your fork to the messages you send your kids with every meal you serve, all the way up to the implications for global-scale stewardship.

You'll feel so virtuous when you finish this chapter that you'll probably have to celebrate with some organic fair-trade chocolate and a pot of rain-forest-preserving herbal tea!

EAT LOCAL (WHEN YOU CAN)

Eating local food is trendy. Once upon a time, everybody ate local food because that was about all they could get. These days, people who choose to eat local, even in the face of a supermarket full of food from other states and even other countries, are called *loca-vores*. Locavores sometimes put very specific requirements on their diets: they will eat only foods that were raised or grown within, say, a fifty-mile radius, or a hundred-mile radius, or in their state, or in their region (such as California or the Midwest or the eastern sea-board). Some are strict, while others allow a few exceptions for a handful of foods they really love, such as coffee (which might be roasted locally), or bananas or avocados or fish.

But you don't have to call yourself a locavore to get all the benefits of this simple return to the good ol' days. You don't have to make any rules about it or be overly restrictive. You can take it as far as you want to take it, and that can mean simply visiting the farmers' market whenever you can and choosing a locally produced food over a nonlocal food when you have the option. Eating more local food is a fantastic way to positively influence a whole chain: Local foods are better for you, your kids, your farmers, your town, the economy, and the whole darned planet!

First of all, local food has to travel a lot shorter distance to get to your dinner plate than food from across the country, not to mention food shipped from other countries. That means the energy spent and the pollution released to transport that food from its point of origin to your dinner plate is *less*. To use the current "green" lingo, local food has a smaller carbon footprint than nonlocal food.

Second, local food is usually fresher exactly because it hasn't spent all those days or weeks on a truck or a boat or however it got to you. Often, local food from the farmers' market was picked the same day you bought it. Yum! It's probably more nutritious too, just because when produce is picked, it immediately begins to lose some of its nutritional power. For example, vitamin C degrades quickly after picking. Local food needs less preserving because it isn't getting bumped around on that truck or boat all week. A lot of produce is coated with wax to prevent damage during shipping, and sometimes it's even picked unripe and gassed to ripen it. Gross.

On top of all that, fresher food just tastes better, so it's more in line with our VIPP (Very Important Pleasure Principle!)

Eating locally also helps you to eat more seasonally. I think it feels better to eat in sync with your climate. For me, that means baby greens, peas, and strawberries in the spring; tomatoes, peppers, melons, and plums in the summer; apples, pears, grapes, and winter squashes in the fall; bitter greens and local meat and eggs in the winter. Without getting too mystical about it, eating seasonally just makes me notice and appreciate the natural world more, and I believe our bodies understand how to digest seasonal foods best. We feel better, and that's worth a million bucks. Plus, back to that whole pleasure thing we Real Moms are so obsessed with: seasonal foods taste best. They're even less expensive! Are we seasonal eaters lucky or what? Sometimes I'll buy extra of something that looks particularly fresh and good, like juicy berries or ripe tomatoes in the summer, and I'll freeze them so I can enjoy them even after the season is over—just for a little reminder of a lovely season that has already passed (and an extra boost of vitamins in produce-starved winter).

If those aren't reasons enough, buying local food from local farmers stimulates your local economy. Every dollar you spend is a vote for something, so spending your dollars at the farmers' market instead of the supermarket sends a message: *I care about my food, I want it fresh, I want it closer to its natural state, I want to support family farms, and I want to keep my money in my own community!* Real Moms, you are so socially *responsible!*

I feel blessed to have so many wonderful farmers' markets near where I live. One of them is a winter market, a trend I'm seeing all over the country. The one near me is called the Green City Market, and it's held inside a huge heated tent, next to the Nature Museum, here in Chicago. It runs from November to April, so I can get food from local farmers any time of year, including not just hothouse-grown fruits and vegetables but also local cheese, meats, poultry, eggs, and even yummy specialty items like homemade baked goods, fresh herbs, and locally made crafts.

But I know not all communities have as many local food resources. You may not have a farmers' market—or do you? Some aren't widely publicized. Ask around to see if anybody knows. If you really don't have a farmer's market, check out your local grocery store or supermarket for local produce. Sometimes it's labeled, or ask the manager. Whole Foods also stocks local food when it can, and so do many health-food stores and food co-ops. Even a roadside stand with fresh watermelons, peaches, apples, or tomatoes can be a great source of local food. Look for them in and around your own community, or even when you travel. I never miss a chance to pick up some local food from wherever I am. Find the closest farmers' market in your area at www.localharvest.org.

You may also have a local farmer who produces beef, lamb, pork, chickens, turkeys, and/or eggs. He or she may not advertise widely or at all, and you might have to just "hear about it" from someone, so ask around. Some of these farmers take orders for, say, a whole hog or lamb or some fraction of a steer; then you pick up your fresh local meat from the processor.

Buying food from local food producers can make a really big difference in your community and in how you feel about your community too. In fact, why not buy more things from locally owned businesses instead of big chain stores and restaurants? My very favorite stores and restaurants are locally owned, often by passionate, creative, unique people who truly believe in what they are doing.

One of my favorite local chefs is Rick Bayless, who recently won the title of Top Chef Master from the TV show *Top Chef Masters*, competing against some of the greatest chefs in the country. Rick runs excellent gourmet Mexican restaurants in Chicago. I interviewed Rick for my PBS TV series, and we discussed how being a farmer is such a noble profession. He has formed a nonprofit organization called Frontera Farmer Foundation, which promotes small, sustainable farms in the Chicago area by providing them with capital development grants. They plan to facilitate a year-round interchange between local farmers and consumers, including chefs, to help make local food what Rick calls "the foundation for sustainable regional cuisine." He went on to say, "Great food, like all art, enhances and reflects a community's vitality, growth, and solidarity. Yet history bears witness that great cuisines spring only from healthy local agriculture." Go, Rick! You're making the world a better place.

However, I have to say I'm no extremist. I don't eat local all the time, because if I did, I would have to quit eating bananas, and tea, and . . . chocolate! And I *like* eating bananas and tea and chocolate! Just eat local when you can—because the food is better in so *many ways*. And when you can't eat local, don't worry about it. Worry is worse for you than a banana shipped to your grocery store from South America. Besides, every bite of local food you eat is a step in the right direction toward supporting your community, eating fresher and healthier, and getting more pleasure out of your food, even if you don't do it all that often.

EAT ORGANIC (WHEN YOU CAN)

People get confused about organic food, and no wonder! One day you'll read that anything less than the USDA organic seal on your food and you're practically poisoning yourself. The next day, you'll hear that organic food isn't worth the extra green because it isn't any more nutritious than the conventional stuff.

Personally, I'm a big supporter of organic food. Yes, I know, it costs more. It may or may not be more nutritious. And sometimes the organic produce at the store doesn't look as good as the conventional.

But do you know why? The conventional stuff is *doused in chemicals* so it doesn't get bruised or bugged. Remember that old Joni Mitchell song, "Big Yellow Taxi"? "Give me spots on my apples, but leave me the birds and the bees, please!" Those pesticides and herbicides and waxy coatings that trap the chemicals and prevent bruises are killing the birds and the bees and *us*. I'd rather eat the natural version, thanks.

I'd also rather vote with my food dollars to support the good, honest work of organic farmers. While there is always controversy and differing opinions, and while some organic farmers may be less ethical than others and try to bend the rules, overall the message they send is a positive one for the planet, all the way up and down the food chain. Organic farmers don't use chemicals, so they don't contribute to the poisoning of the planet. Organic farmers are required by law to treat animals humanely (even if the occasional one doesn't), and they aim to protect the soil, water, and animal life for years to come. In my next life, I want to be an organic farmer!

I'm no Pollyanna, even if I do tend to be a bright-eyed optimist. No system is perfect, but the occasional bad-seed organic farm doesn't mean you trash the concept. Buying and eating organic means you put fewer pesticides and other noxious chemicals into that beautiful body of yours, and into the pure and perfect bodies of your children. Is there any better reason to spend an extra two bucks on that bag of apples, even if they don't look perfect enough for a magazine cover?

I also understand that, as with politics and breast-feeding, you don't want to be telling people what to do, unless they ask you (or buy your book). But you're reading my book, so pardon me while I proselytize a bit more. Some foods are just dirtier than others, and I don't mean they are covered with nice, fresh natural soil. I mean they are doused in chemicals. As of the publication of this book, the Organic Consumers Association states that these are the current "dirty dozen" foods most likely to be contaminated with pesticides, herbicides, and other nasties. If you want to eat clean, you can get rid of most of the chemicals in your diet if you *always* buy organic versions of these twelve foods:

1. Peaches
2. Apples
3. Sweet bell peppers
4. Celery
5. Nectarines
6. Strawberries
7. Cherries
8. Pears
9. Imported grapes (grown in U.S. are much better)
10. Spinach
11. Lettuce
12. Potatoes

There's another easy way to find out the level of toxins in your "conventional" produce. The Pesticide Action Network's online database, called "What's on my Food?" compares organic to conventional food and explains exactly what you're eating and drinking. Go to www.WhatsOnMyFood.org and simply click on the food of your choice to find out which pesticides have been used on it. The site is very informative; it explains pesticide toxicity, health impacts of pesticides on the body, and which foods are most likely to include chemicals. Another good site is www.foodnews.org. Yes, obsessively browsing these sorts of Web sites is how I like to spend my leisure time. (I never said I wasn't weird!)

I once interviewed Nell Newman, daughter of Paul Newman, on my PBS TV series. Nell is an organic food guru and author of a great book called *The Newman's Own Organics Guide to a Good Life: Simple Measures That Benefit You and the Place You Live.* In addition to those impressive credentials, she's also a warmhearted and deeply ethical woman.

On the show, I asked Nell what she would tell someone at home wondering whether organic food was worth buying. This is what she said:

> *Well, think about conventional agriculture and think about how things are really grown. They use pesticides to kill the bugs, they use herbicides to kill the weeds, they use fungicides to kill everything in the soil—and those are poisons. So to me it just makes sense. I would rather eat food that has not been poisoned. . . . That's why I choose to eat organic.*

Nell had more to say, specifically about another big issue in organics these days: GMOs, or genetically modified organisms. I asked her to clarify what these were, and she said, "Genetic engineering is something that's done in a lab where you take genetic material from one thing, maybe a frog, and put it in a cabbage."

I joked, "So if your cabbage starts hopping off your plate, you might know why, right?" Silly, but in a way, it's disturbingly close to the reality. Nell added:

> *The concern with genetic engineering is that it's an inexact science and we are not quite sure what the effects are on crops when you introduce a gene from something else. How does that really affect the crop? It probably has many applications in terms of science, but in terms of agriculture it's been let out of the lab, into the field, and genetic engineering is very different than pesticides.*

At least pesticides degrade over time, but genetically engineered crops continue to grow and crossbreed with other crops and contaminate the environment and other crops and other weeds and native plants. That's a great concern. . . . The only thing you can really do is to support organic agriculture, because organic agriculture is the only form of agriculture that doesn't allow genetic engineering.

Well said, Nell! I couldn't agree with you more.

TAKE A LOOK AT YOUR TRASH

Even the purest, most organic food in the world isn't as earth-friendly as it could be if it's all sealed up in a plastic tray covered by a plastic wrapper covered by a cardboard box wrapped in more plastic.

Another one of my big platforms (I have a lot of those, and I don't mean platform shoes!) is trash. Trash, trash, trash. We Americans generate an obscene amount of trash, and it's clogging up our landfills and oceans. We're filling up our dear Mother Earth with the refuse of our consumerism-obsessed existences (to be a bit poetic about it)!

If this bugs you the way it bugs me, there are some things you can do. First, recycle! Many communities have curbside recycling, and if yours does, this is such an easy way to add less to landfills. Every time you throw something away, stop for two seconds to consider whether it could be recycled. If you aren't sure, call up your city or county or whoever recycles in your area, and ask them. Many have recycling guides they can send you. Or if you don't have curbside recycling, make your own bin for cardboard, paper, glass, aluminum, and plastics, and cart them off to a local recycling center once a week, when you are already out and about running errands.

Recycled items are used to make other products, so not only does your aluminum can or plastic bottle *not* go into a landfill, but it reduces the need to manufacture more materials to make more products. It's doubly ecofriendly.

Another thing I consider when buying a packaged product is the nature of the packaging itself. I prefer to buy products in packages that are not only recyclable, but already recycled. These might be made of cardboard, paper, plastic, or glass. Again, you're voting with your dollars to buy products that use discarded materials instead of making new materials. Score another one for Mother Earth!

Some recycled packaging is really creative. It might be made from corn or soy, or old soda bottles. Or it might be made from sustainable crops that don't deplete the environment, like hemp. It's amazing what you can find out if you ask a few questions and read the labels.

As with organics, the recycling system isn't perfect. The system is definitely prone to greenwashing, that nasty trend wherein manufacturers try to make their products look greener than they really are, just to cash in on the trend. However, recycling is definitely a step in the right direction. It doesn't take that much time, and it's not that much trouble, for a potentially huge impact on the environment.

However, there is something even better you can do when it comes to trash: Make less. We've taken a few mini steps in our home to reduce trash, and the results have been major. We make just a fraction of the trash we used to make. I look for minimally packaged products, but even better, I use the bulk bins in my grocery store. You can hugely reduce your trash load by scooping your rice, quinoa, pumpkin seeds, granola, nuts, lentils, etc., straight from a bulk bin into a paper or plastic bag yourself. You write the number of the bin onto a sticker or twist-tie, and then the cashier weighs your bag at the register. Some stores even have scales so you can weigh it yourself and print out a handy label. Easy-peasy!

I buy most of my staple foods in bulk, and transfer them into glass containers when I get home. Frankly, this will get you eating more whole foods too. Two Real Mom concepts accomplished in one easy act? Score!

At my local food cooperative, I can skip the plastic bags entirely by bringing, for example, my oats container (in my cloth bag) to the shop, weighing the container before I fill it to get what's called "tare weight," and then pouring the oats from the bulk container straight into my own container. At the checkout counter, the tare weight is deducted from the whole before I'm charged per pound. I do this for maple syrup, quinoa, rice, and wheat germ, which reduces the number of little plastic bags that cycle through my kitchen (although the plain plastic bags by the bulk bin are still much preferable to conventional packaging, because they're not printed on and machine sealed, all of which costs the planet time, energy, and resources).

Skip the bags for your produce and just lay it gently in your grocery cart, or bring a box or bag from home. Don't forget your cloth grocery bags, either—rather than having to mull over the "paper or plastic" question, you'll be set with your own eco-friendly option. I especially like the ChicoBags that fold up into a handy pouch with a clip. I just clip one on my purse and I am always ready with a bag.

When you bring your own shopping bags, you usually get a tiny discount per bag, and you won't have to try to figure out where to store those seven zillion plastic grocery bags somewhere in your kitchen (you know you have that one drawer or cabinet full of them, right?). It never hurts to have a few of them around—I leave two in my car, for unexpected shopping trips, and they are good for wet towels and bathing suits after a day at the pool or beach with the kids—but you really don't need to be bringing more home every week.

We're a bit behind the times in the United States in terms of bags at the market. A friend told me that when she was food shopping in Italy twenty years ago, the clerk added a charge onto her grocery bill for the plastic bags the store provided! And I just heard from another friend of mine who lives in California; the state is considering banning plastic grocery bags entirely, since those bags are not biodegradable and take up space in landfills for a long, long time (something like a thousand years!). They may also charge five cents per paper bag for shoppers who forgot their own bags. Can you imagine if every one of us Real Moms made that one small change and lugged our own bags to the market? What an amazing, profound impact we'd make.

In other words, whenever you can avoid packaging of any kind, go for it!

Maybe someday all this will be unnecessary. (There I go, donning my rose-colored glasses again—but I think they make me look fabulous.) Lots of food companies are reducing their packaging because we Real Moms have complained and requested and begged and cajoled them into it. They are beginning to recognize that less packaging makes good economic sense. When green is profitable, it will take over the world! Request less packaging from your grocers, and if they hear it enough, they'll respond.

One more thing you might want to consider seriously: composting. If you garden or you just want to make your trees and shrubs healthier, consider creating a small pile in an out-of-the-way corner of your yard for plant food scraps, grass clippings, and raked leaves. Stir it up every so often and in about a year you've got black gold that is like a magic bullet for anything growing in your yard. I've read that Americans throw away almost half of the food produced in this country, and it costs about one billion dollars annually to send all that food waste to landfills, where it decomposes and creates methane, a greenhouse gas that captures heat in the atmosphere as carbon dioxide. Composting keeps that food waste out of landfills and in your own backyard, literally!

Now that we've got that straight, take a moment and decide whether or not your daily consumption is depleting our natural resources. My daily goal is to maintain balance and use only what I can replace. It's a tricky task, but if you shoot for perfect and you miss, you're still doing a great job. Real Moms live in the real world, and if we all did the best we could, we'd all be better off.

And when you do find yourself with some extra plastic packaging hanging around, or a few extra plastic bags, for heaven's sake, don't pitch them into the trash. There are times when I do have to purchase food in plastic containers at the store. When I do, I use up the food inside, wash out the container, and save it. I have a small stack in my pantry so that when guests come over for dinner, I can send them home with a recyclable plastic food container of leftovers. Recycling mission accomplished!

GO VEG (WHEN YOU CAN)

Just to set the record straight, I am not a vegetarian. I love a juicy steak as much as the next gal. However, I do know that factory farming is questionable in terms of its treatment of animals (some might say horrific). I don't like that. It bothers me. It makes me feel uncomfortable, and I don't like feeling uncomfortable. Worse yet, recent often-quoted research shows that animal agriculture contributes more greenhouse gases than all the cars in the world. *In the world!* Yikes.

I eat meat, but I have been convinced by the many nutritionists and doctors I studied with at the Institute for Integrative Nutrition that grass-fed meat is much healthier for the body. Grass-fed cows are eating a diet much more suited to their natures, so their meat is healthier. Factory-farmed animals that are fed an unnatural diet of corn and who knows what else develop numerous health problems—and then we eat them? And feed them to our children?

I am a firm believer that a diet rich in fruits and vegetables with just a little bit of grass-fed beef, poultry raised in a barnyard with time in the sunshine, and wild-caught fish (the kinds that aren't endangered) make the best possible diet. Add delicious whole grains, cut out most of the white flour, white sugar, and trans fat, and you're good to go. In fact, I can practically guarantee that you will begin to *glow*.

But we can all use a day or two off meat every week.

Going veg once or twice a week can make a huge difference in your health, your digestion, your complexion, and your energy. It also impacts the environment. If you eat less meat and processed foods, you'll eat more fruits, vegetables, and whole grains. It's just math. Choose high-quality meat, poultry, and seafood, even if it costs more (you get what you pay for), but eat it less often. You'll be doing the right thing by your body, and you'll reduce your contribution to pollution-spewing animal agriculture, and that is doing the right thing by the planet.

About Milk

ONE OF MY dear friends told me a story about how she once visited a new friend and caught a glimpse inside the refrigerator. "Where's the milk?" she asked in surprise, wondering how anyone could have breakfast without milk.

Her host said, "Where have you been?" and then began to educate her. At that time, my friend had never met a vegetarian or vegan, had never thought about the politics of animal protein or the quality of life of the cows and chickens and pigs she was eating, and certainly hadn't known anything about bovine growth hormone, the hormone they pump into dairy cows in the United States to make them produce more milk, or the unnatural grain-based diet they eat, or all the antibiotics they give dairy cows because of the constant breast infections they get from overproducing. Ouch.

She had always been a big milk drinker, thinking it was a healthy dietary choice, until that moment. From then on, she vowed to keep a milk-free refrigerator as well. She knew enough to understand that hormones that amp up a lactating cow's milk production coupled with stray antibiotics were not ingredients she wanted on her breakfast menu.

Fortunately, some dairies produce milk without these growth hormones and antibiotics. Organic milk may not contain them, either. So the next time you are grabbing that jug off the shelf, think about the state of the jugs from whence it came . . . and you might think twice. So organic milk is an extra two bucks? Sounds like a bargain to me.

But I'm also a firm believer in living by your firm beliefs. For some Real Moms, it's never okay to eat an animal, and that's fine too. A totally vegetarian diet, or even a vegan diet (no eggs, dairy, honey, or anything else that comes from an animal), can be a very healthy way to eat, as long as you stick to your resolve to eat less white flour, sugar, and trans fat, because even though those nasty substances don't contain animal fat, they don't contain anything good for you, either. If your beliefs center more around the overall health of the planet, it just makes sense to have a meatless dinner a few times a week or more, and to choose grass-fed organic beef from small family farms when you do eat it.

I also believe each woman is different. Some need more meat than others. Some love fish and some think it's creepy. Some need a little more convincing than others to eat their daily dose of fruits and veggies. But think about this: What you *prefer* isn't necessarily the same as what makes you *feel best*. You've probably heard someone (maybe it was you!) say something along the lines of, "Oh, I love cheeseburgers, but they sure don't love me!" Pay attention to your *inner environment* when making your food choices. You can be inner-ecofriendly in your dietary choices too. If meat makes you feel heavy and tired, eat less of it, even if you like it. If a little meat gives you a much-needed feeling of well-being, then have some. You don't have to cut it out of your life entirely. Just go easy. Moderation is almost always the best course.

The bottom line is that going veg is a personal decision, but there is no question that eating *less* meat and choosing higher-*quality* meat that doesn't come from a large-scale animal agriculture machine is a cleaner, purer, healthier, and greener choice.

BY THE WAY, YOU'RE BEING WATCHED

In case you haven't noticed . . . someone is spying on you. Everything you say, everything you do, practically everything you *think* is being recorded. No, not on a tape recorder—in your children's brains! Kids watch everything, and every action you take is being programmed into their very being. It's true. Have you ever seen your child "doing" your behavior? You are more powerful and influential than you ever imagined you would be.

My husband has a certain gesture he makes with his eyebrows, and the other day, my son did it too. It's so subconscious, they probably don't even realize they're doing it. And you *know* you've caught yourself in the mirror or in a shop window looking *exactly like* one of your parents, or heard something come out of your mouth only your mother would say, or making that silly over-the-top hand gesture your dad always makes. And your parents probably do things they got from their parents. It's just the way of the world. Don't even pretend it hasn't happened to you!

Considering, then, your newly realized, almost supernatural influence, it only makes good sense to start (or continue) good habits that are mindful, compassionate, and reflect care of other people, animals, and the planet. An obvious way to state this is the old saying, "Children do what you do, not what you say." When you act kindly, compassionately, and with care toward others, your children will learn that. When you express your delight with fruits and vegetables, your children will learn that. When you vocalize your disgust with pesticides on crops and processed foods filled with chemicals and junk like high-fructose corn syrup and white flour, your children will learn that too. If you go to the farmers' market, so will they. If you bring your own bag to the market, they'll come to believe that's the right thing to do. Sure, they may not do it now. They may roll their eyes or scoff at you (especially if they are teenagers), but think about this: No matter how they rebel, most kids come back around to their parents' point of view in the end. When it counts—when they inherit the earth, as the next generation inevitably will—they will have the tools they need to keep this planet spinning along, happily populated with healthy people.

Many times after playdates, the mothers of my sons' friends have told me, "Your son is such a good eater, and so polite!" I blush and then think, *Well, of course! I'm a good eater, and I think I'm pretty polite too.* I say thank-you for the compliment and then I smile as I mentally pat myself on the back. And so should you when someone compliments *your* child—the apple surely doesn't fall far from the tree, and you should be proud of that! In fact, I think you should reward yourself with some chocolate.

I know—again with the chocolate? But I have a good excuse to bring it up again. When you purchase chocolate marked as Rainforest Alliance Certified, you know the cocoa is sustainably harvested. You can support the preservation of the rain forest *and* eat chocolate. Can you believe it? Virtue in a chocolate bar? That's the kind of ecofriendly I can *really* get behind! Tell your friends!

DO FIVE THINGS

This week, it's all about your ethics and how they fit or don't fit into the way you eat the food you love. So let's flex those I-care muscles. Here are the five things I'd like you to do this week:

1. GO TO YOUR LOCAL FARMERS' MARKET AND PURCHASE AT LEAST ONE LOCALLY PRODUCED VEGETABLE OR FRUIT. TALK TO THE FARMER AND GET TO KNOW THE SOURCE OF YOUR FOOD.

Look for what's in season, and ask exactly where it was grown. Ask about the farm and what this year's growing season was like. Ask about the best ways to prepare the food you want to buy. Get the *story* behind the food. You'll be able to take it home and appreciate it more when you serve it for dinner.

2. SWITCH AT LEAST THREE FOODS IN YOUR PANTRY/REFRIGERATOR TO ORGANIC.

I hope you'll choose some from the dirty-dozen list in this chapter. Better yet, swap out *all* the foods from the dirty dozen that you tend to eat and serve to your family, and try organic milk if your kids drink a lot of it. Go organic and feel *clean.*

3. LOOK AT THE PACKAGING ON YOUR FOOD. IS IT EARTH-FRIENDLY?

The next time you go to the store, keep packaging in mind. Look for indications that the product's packaging is both recycled and recyclable. Keep sending the stuff around so we don't have to make any more plastic, paper, or glass.

4. GO VEG ONCE A WEEK . . . THEN TWICE.

Do it for your body, do it for your soul, do it for the animals, and do it for the planet. You don't have to go all the way. Just go a *little* bit of the way. I'm talking second base, tops. It will make a big difference, I promise.

5. THANK GOODNESS YOU'RE STILL DRINKING YOUR EIGHT GLASSES OF FRESH, PURE WATER EVERY DAY!

If you're getting bored, get reinspired by watching the movie *Flow*, about the world water crisis. Fascinating! Find out more about it at www.flowthefilm.com.

Wow. Can you believe it? Ten weeks just *flew by*, if you ask me. What a great ride. I bet you're feeling absolutely fantastic. I know I am! Before you head straight into part three of this book, I'd like you to look back through the first ten chapters and think back over the last ten weeks since you started the RMLTE plan. Which habits have stuck with you? Which didn't work so well? I would never expect you to adopt every single tidbit of advice in this book, but I hope you've discovered some great new ideas and healthy habits that have changed your life, even just a little. Take the ones close to your heart, embrace them, and make them part of your life. Those that didn't stick, well . . . keep them in the back of your mind, and maybe you'll come back around to them later.

After you've mulled this over, dig into part three for more structure and inspiration—it contains three weeks' worth of meals and recipes I just know you're going to love. Follow it precisely if you are that kind of person, or just pick out the parts that get you excited, if you are *that* kind of person. I offer these recipes to you with love, gratitude, and the healthy glow that comes from living clean and loving food—I wish I could give you all the biggest hug! So on that note, *bon appétit*, cheers, and may all Real Moms learn how to love themselves with the same passion and fervor with which they love their children.

PART THREE

Happy Endings:

The *Real Moms Love to Eat* Plan in Practice

Time to Eat!

NOW THE *REAL* fun begins!

In this final section, all of the elements we've talked about throughout the book come together into a three-week daily meal plan, complete with irresistible recipes. You can be as strict or as freewheeling as you like with this plan. Incorporate the good habits you've picked up in parts one and two, and if I include a food that makes you go, "Eww," then for goodness' sake, don't eat it! Replace it with something you love that's similar in amount, type, and nutrient balance (for example, substitute an apple for a banana—but *not* for a quarter-pound slice of apple pastry or banana cake with frosting!).

This twenty-one-day meal plan is specifically designed to help *feed you*, so you have not just the satisfaction of good food, but more energy and vitality. It will help bring out your sparkle. I also hope it will inspire you to get into your kitchen and start making your meals out of whole foods. You'll be cementing the habits you've learned in this book into your daily life, as your love affair with food grows into a long-term relationship.

The more you eat well, to please and nourish your body, mind, and soul, the sooner you will begin to enjoy a lifetime of vibrant health, glowing good looks, nutritional intelligence, and yes, some serious sex appeal. And those extra pounds? They're about to start melting away, girlfriend. They are practically *ancient history*.

Go ahead and mix and match elements from each day, making this plan your own. As long as you maintain the integrity of the plan's basic structure, you should be fine. Throughout the first twenty-one days of the plan, relish the taste of everything you eat. Eat slowly, and really savor each bite. Let your taste buds run wild with flavor—the sweetness of dried fruit, the saltiness of pickles, the sourness of citrus, and the crisp bitterness of leafy greens. Every single bite has the potential to thrill you.

Taste things one at a time, or enjoy them entwined with one another. Take note of how they impact one another. You'll refine your palate, amp up your pleasure, and be teaching your kids the importance of healthy food, all at the same time. What could be sweeter?

A few notes before we launch:

* Menu items with recipes to follow are marked with an *. When the recipe appears earlier in the book, I'll reference the page number for you.

* Remember the concept of cooking once, eating two or three times. If you can't finish your meal, or you prepare extra, save it and enjoy it again tomorrow rather than making something new. You won't always want to cook. I've incorporated suggestions for doing this throughout—when I want you to set aside something for a meal the next day (a piece of salmon, a bit of salad, a serving of soup), I'll let you know.

* Keep drinking that water! It's your own personal fountain of youthful energy.

* I would never tell you to give up your comforting morning cuppa—this plan allows for up to two cups of coffee or freshly brewed tea each day, which I won't bother to mention again. Indulge if that's *you*. You can even add a teaspoon of organic cream, soy creamer, rice milk, local honey, or stevia, if you so desire. You can have as much noncaffeinated herbal tea as you like. It's another great way to stay hydrated.

* The meals in this plan average out to about two thousand calories a day, more or less (based on loose but not technical estimates). This plan is definitely *not* about undereating, but it's not about overeating either. You may think two thousand calories sounds like a lot, but most people actually eat more without even realizing it, especially snacking mindlessly in front of the TV or helping themselves to seconds at dinner. Ironically, people on diets tend to eat more, when they think they are eating less, because the deprivation makes them overeat in the evenings or every few days, and the sum total may average out to much more than two thousand calories per day. In this plan, every bite counts, and you'll get all the nutrition you need. You won't feel deprived or hungry—just satisfied, pleasured, and *alive*.

* I keep telling you that you can modify this plan to suit you—and I really mean it!—but no matter how you do it, make sure you eat plenty of fruits and vegetables. It's the best thing you can do for yourself. The government may recommend five servings a day, but healthy humans should really be eating ten to twelve servings a day. Add them to anything and everything whenever you get the chance.

* Try to eat at least every three to four hours, so you never get to the point where you are ravenous and ready to eat the tablecloth.

* Each day of the plan will include notes, a menu, and some recipes for breakfast, a midmorning snack, lunch, an afternoon snack, and dinner. Many days include an optional dessert. You can eat an optional dessert every day if you really want one. Any of the dessert recipes in this section or earlier in the book will do. Just keep your portion small and savor every bite!

* I also couldn't help tossing in a few sexy lifestyle tips to help you reduce stress, get moving, and feel better about yourself. Keep an eye out for those inspirational boxes.

* Many of the recipes in this section of the book were contributed by friends, colleagues, and mentors of mine. You can find out more about them in the Helpful People part of the Resources section at the back of this book.

THE EATING PLAN

DAY ONE

Ready to start feeling like a sexy mama? Because you are*! Really enjoy your food today—that's what it's all about.*

Breakfast

- ► Green Smoothie*
- ► Hard-boiled egg, sliced and seasoned with a dash of sea salt and/or cracked pepper

GREEN SMOOTHIE

■ **SERVES 1.**

I've already given you a couple of smoothie recipes, but here's another one, a variation I often make based on the one from Karyn's Raw Café and store in Chicago. Karyn makes her own raw Karyn's Green Meal Powder and it's my go-to green powder for smoothies, superquick and simple. I often include coconut water in this smoothie—it's low in carbs, fats, and sugars and carries nutrients and oxygen to cells. Purchase soy lecithin granules at any health-food or natural-food store, such as Whole Foods Market or Trader Joe's. Soy lecithin helps oils, fats, and water combine more smoothly in your smoothie.

8 ounces pure organic apple juice (or 4 ounces apple juice and 4 ounces coconut water)
1 heaping tablespoon Karyn's Green Meal Powder or powdered greens of your choice (available in health-food stores) or a huge handful of mixed greens from the garden or the farmers' market, when they are in season

1 teaspoon soy lecithin granules
1 tablespoon flaxseed oil or other omega fatty acid oil (I like
   Udo's 3-6-9 Oil)
1 frozen banana
1 tablespoon freshly ground flaxseeds
1 scoop vanilla whey or hemp protein (right now, I'm loving
   rBGH-free Tera's Whey. It's tasty and clean)

Blend all of the ingredients on a low speed until creamy. Enjoy with a green mustache!

Midmorning Snack

▸ 1 small container of plain or vanilla low-sugar or sugar-free yogurt topped with ¼ cup high-fiber cereal, like Kashi Organic Promise Autumn Wheat, and 5 to 8 chopped almonds and blueberries. You can also choose plain yogurt. If it's not sweet enough, try a tiny pinch of stevia (a little goes a long way), or add a dash of cinnamon and a spoonful of honey or agave nectar. Tasty!

▸ I also love Lifeway Kefir, a high-calcium, high-protein, yogurt-style beverage. My favorite flavor is the Chocolate Truffle (what a shocker, right?).

FEED YOUR SOUL:
Midmorning Gratitude Break

BEFORE YOUR MIDMORNING snack, take a minute, close your eyes, and slowly breathe in and out through your nose. Now open your eyes and say, "Thank you." Go ahead, say it out loud! It's a snack for your soul.

Lunch

▶ Huge Salad*

HUGE SALAD

■ **SERVES 1.**

The easiest way to get all those beauty-enhancing, energy-bestowing, immune-building vegetables into your daily diet is to have a salad with every lunch and dinner. For lunch, I love a big salad with some protein. Nobody says you can't put it in a big mixing bowl. The more greens and raw veggies the better, so get creative. Add a little lean protein and you are good to go. Mix your own dressing and skip the croutons to avoid unnecessary, energy-zapping simple carbs. If this makes too much, just save the rest to have as a side salad for dinner.

4 cups mixed greens
3 ounces grilled salmon or chicken breast (leftovers from last night's dinner are fine too)
2 cups chopped raw vegetables, such as broccoli, cauliflower, bell peppers, shredded carrots, chopped celery, sliced radishes, or whatever else is fresh and in season
1 pear, sliced

Toss everything together in a big bowl and drizzle with 2 tablespoons of your favorite dressing. Better yet, make your own Italian dressing: whisk together ¼ cup balsamic vinegar, ½ cup extra virgin olive oil, 1 teaspoon agave nectar, 1 teaspoon dried crushed Italian seasoning (or a pinch each of dried oregano, basil, and thyme), sea salt, and freshly ground black pepper to taste, and, optionally, 1 minced garlic clove. This makes more than one serving—remember, just drizzle it on. Two tablespoons max.

Afternoon Snack

- 2 tablespoons natural nut butter (I like Justin's individually packaged nut butters in all their great flavors) on 1 apple, sliced, or 3 stalks of celery. Who says it's just for kids? I love this snack.

FEED YOUR BODY:
Posture Nudge

SIT WITH YOUR back perfectly straight, stretching your shoulder blades back toward each other. Reach back behind you with both arms straight and grasp your hands together near your tush, interlacing your fingers. Gently pull your clasped hands up for an easy shoulder stretch. Don't pull hard; just give your shoulders a nice gentle stretch.

Dinner

- Superfast Pureed White Bean Soup with Leeks and Carrots*

- Lime-crusted Spiced Salmon*

- Leftover salad from lunch

Both of these dinner recipes come from my talented friend Ivy Larson, the author of three healthy-living books (including *The Gold Coast Cure*). She currently works as a healthy-living coach and runs the www.CleanCuisine.com Web site. Ivy was a wonderful guest on my radio show; her energy is contagious. Maybe it's the food?

SUPERFAST PUREED WHITE BEAN SOUP WITH LEEKS AND CARROTS

■ SERVES 4.

3 tablespoons extra virgin olive oil
2 whole leek stalks, sliced into thin rounds
Sea salt, to taste
White pepper, to taste
4 cloves garlic, minced
2 whole carrots, peeled and chopped
2 cans (19 ounces each) organic cannellini beans, rinsed and
    drained
Juice from 1 whole lemon
3 cups organic vegetable broth (such as Pacific Natural Foods)
¼ cup chopped parsley

1. Heat the oil over medium-high heat in a large soup pot. Add the leeks and sauté, stirring often, for 2 to 3 minutes, or until they just begin to soften. Season leeks with salt and white pepper to taste. Add the garlic and carrots; cook for an additional 2 to 3 minutes.

2. Add the beans, lemon juice and vegetable broth. Simmer for 3 to 4 minutes. Add the parsley. Use a handheld immersion blender to process soup into a creamy puree (or puree a little bit at a time in a regular blender, but be careful blending hot soup!). Season with salt and pepper to taste. Serve warm, as a side to the salmon below (save 1 serving leftover soup for tomorrow's lunch).

LIME-CRUSTED SPICED SALMON

■ SERVES 4.

Extra virgin olive oil (to grease the pan)
1½ pounds wild salmon fillets

½ teaspoon Old Bay Seasoning
½ teaspoon dried basil
¼ teaspoon Jamaican curry powder (optional)
2 teaspoons lime zest (grated from a fresh organic lime)
½ cup whole-wheat panko crumbs (such as Ian's Natural Foods)
1 tablespoon cold organic grass-fed butter, sliced into very thin
pieces
Juice from 1 whole lime

1. Preheat oven to 375 degrees. Lightly oil a 9"-x-11" baking dish with extra virgin olive oil.

2. Place salmon in the baking dish. Sprinkle with Old Bay Seasoning, dried basil, Jamaican curry powder, and lime zest. Sprinkle panko crumbs on top. Dot the butter on top of salmon. Place salmon in the oven and bake for 15 minutes.

3. Remove salmon from the oven; squeeze lime juice on top. Let stand 2 to 3 minutes before serving. Serve warm. (Save one piece of salmon for tomorrow—tastes great cold on top of a salad!)

DAY TWO

Today you'll get lots of great protein. Take advantage of the fact by getting some exercise—or lifting small children into the air. And-a-one, and-a-two, and-a-three. How many reps can you do with a toddler?

Breakfast

► Two scrambled eggs with lightly steamed broccoli and/ or asparagus. I like to mix 3 tablespoons of rice milk into my scrambled eggs to make them fluffy, along with a dash of sea salt and cracked black pepper.

► Sliced fruit (because something about slicing fruit just makes it taste better, but if you like your fruit whole or you're on the go, just eat the equivalent of one piece of whole fruit)

Midmorning Snack

- ▶ Green Smoothie* (Use the recipe from yesterday on page 198, but add ¼ cup frozen berries for an extra dose of antioxidants)
- ▶ Rudi's Organic Bakery multigrain English muffin with flax and a schmear of organic strawberry jam

FEED YOUR BODY:
Midmorning Rejuvenation

STAND UP, WHEREVER you are. Bring your chin to your chest and then slowly roll down your spine, head and arms relaxed and hanging loosely, toward the floor. Can you touch your toes? If not, do this every day until you can. Don't push, don't bounce, don't strain. This should feel *delicious*. Hang there for thirty seconds and then slowly roll up in reverse order.

Lunch

- ▶ Balsamic Broccoli Salad*
- ▶ Salmon and/or soup left over from yesterday's dinner

BALSAMIC BROCCOLI SALAD

■ SERVES 4.

This recipe comes from Ivy Larson.

1 head fresh broccoli, cut into bite-size pieces
5 to 6 garlic cloves, minced

¼ cup balsamic vinegar
2 tablespoons flaxseed, hemp, or extra virgin olive oil
A pinch of dried oregano (or to taste)
Sea salt, to taste
Black pepper, to taste

1. Prepare an ice bath by filling a large bowl with ice and water. Bring several inches of water to a boil in a large covered pot. Add the broccoli to the boiling water; cook 3 to 4 minutes (or until just tender when pierced with a fork). Drain immediately. Plunge broccoli into ice bath for 2 minutes.

2. Drain broccoli again and lightly pat dry with paper towels. Place broccoli in a large bowl. Add the garlic, balsamic vinegar, oil, and oregano. Season with salt and pepper, to taste. Chill the broccoli in the freezer for 10 to 15 minutes or in the refrigerator for 30 minutes. Serve cold.

Afternoon Snack

▶ Eric the Trainer's Protein Bomb*

FEED YOUR MIND AND BODY:
Real Moms Love Protein!

TAKE A MOMENT and give thanks for the strength and vitality you will receive from the beautiful protein-rich snack you are about to eat.

🍳 ERIC THE TRAINER'S PROTEIN BOMB!

■ **SERVES 2 TO 3.**

1 can dolphin-safe tuna (find a brand made in America—more humane!)
1 small container organic cottage cheese (about 1 cup)
1 cup fresh sliced pineapple (you can buy pineapple precut in the store)
½ cup fresh pico de gallo (buy in the deli section, or chop and combine 1 tomato, ½ small white onion, one garlic clove, ½ bell pepper, and optionally ½ jalapeno pepper. Add juice from one fresh lime and a sprinkle of fresh cilantro)

Cut the pineapple into small, bite-size pieces. Put in a bowl and combine with the cottage cheese. Spread this mixture onto a plate. Flake tuna with a fork, then sprinkle on top of cottage cheese mixture. Top with pico de gallo, and enjoy an exotic mixture of protein-building perfection!

Dinner

▶ Watermelon, Pistachio and Baby Greens Salad (with Rock Shrimp)*

🍳 WATERMELON, PISTACHIO AND BABY GREENS SALAD (WITH ROCK SHRIMP)

■ **SERVES 4 TO 6.**

I love this delightful salad created by my friend Sarah Copeland, writer (www.edibleliving.com), urban gardener, passionate cook, and curator of good living. By day, she is a seasoned recipe developer; by night, a consummate forager for edible adventures.

Rock shrimp has a flavor akin to lobster but cooks like regular shrimp to deliver a fast punch of protein to this otherwise light and lively salad. This is the perfect salad to show off your windowsill or backyard garden of summer greens. The secret to this salad's bright flavor is the variety of textures and tastes that come from the different kinds of greens and herbs—soft, buttery butter lettuce, punchy arugula, and tender mâche or purslane pop with the garnish of fresh mint, chives, and coarse sea salt. All together, with the watermelon and the luscious healthy fats of olive oil, it plays to your desires for sweet and salty, fresh and buttery, with utterly vibrant satisfaction.

1 lb. rock shrimp
1 tablespoon olive oil
¼ teaspoon cayenne pepper
½ teaspoon sea salt
¼ teaspoon black pepper
2 small heads butter lettuce, torn
2 heaping handfuls young arugula
1 heaping handful mâche, purslane, or watercress
½ medium seedless watermelon, rind removed and cut in wedges
¼ cup mint, peppermint, or spearmint leaves, torn
1 teaspoon chopped chives
Coarse white, gray, or pink sea salt
Freshly ground black pepper
4 tablespoons finest extra virgin olive oil, or to taste
½ lemon
¼ cup pistachios

1. Lay shrimp on a lined surface and use a paring knife to split slightly down the back to help it cook evenly. Toss the shrimp with the oil, cayenne, salt, and pepper in a large bowl. Leave shrimp in the fridge to marinate while you prepare the salad.

2. Arrange the lettuce on a platter. Distribute the arugula and mâche, purslane, or watercress and watermelon wedges over the top. Garnish the salad with the radishes, torn mint and chives, and season liberally with sea salt. Drizzle to your taste with your finest extra virgin olive oil.

3. To finish, heat a medium pan over medium-high heat. Add the shrimp to the hot pan and cook, stirring until every shrimp is just pink throughout. Turn off the heat; squeeze the lemon over the top to release all the good bits from the pan and make a light, flavorful sauce. Top the salad with the rock shrimp and spoon cooking juices over the top like a dressing. Sprinkle with pistachios and serve.

DAY THREE

I'm so excited that we're making Energy Kale Salad today. I could probably eat it every single day for lunch. I hope you love it as much as I do! This is a high-energy-food day, so go for a brisk walk.

Breakfast

▶ Peanut Butter Chocolate Green Smoothie. Use Green Smoothie recipe from day one except substitute almond or rice milk for apple juice and add:

- 1 tablespoon of natural, unsweetened organic peanut butter (or other nut butter of your choice)
- 1 tablespoon raw cacao powder
- 1 tablespoon raw agave nectar (optional)

▶ **OPTIONAL:** Poached egg with sea salt, if you are still hungry (but that smoothie may be more than enough!)

Midmorning Snack

▶ Clif Bar, LUNA Bar, or other favorite protein bar. I love both of these bars because I can throw them in my purse and pull them out anywhere—no utensils needed. They are a good source of protein, fiber, and carbohydrates.

▶ ½ cup fresh cherries—on the go, bring a zipper bag to capture the pits

Lunch

- ▶ Energy Kale Salad*
- ▶ 2 to 4 Mini Turkey Meatballs, cold (buy premade from store or make the recipe that follows)*
- ▶ **OPTIONAL:** 1 tablespoon ketchup or barbecue sauce

ENERGY KALE SALAD

■ **SERVES 4 TO 6.**

The first time my friend Bonita made her kale salad for me, I licked the plate! Seriously. It's that good.

1 bunch of lacinato kale (also known as dinosaur kale, or use
   any other kind of kale)
1 green zucchini diced into ⅛-inch cubes
½ red onion diced into ⅛-inch cubes
Juice of 1 lemon (about 3 tablespoons)
3 tablespoons olive oil
¼ teaspoon ground cumin
⅛ teaspoon cayenne pepper
¼ teaspoon sea salt
⅛ teaspoon black pepper

1. Remove center stems from each kale leaf. Chop kale into thin ribbons (by rolling it up and slicing as thinly as you can). Add it to a large bowl along with the diced zucchini and onions.

2. In separate bowl, whisk together lemon juice, olive oil, cumin, cayenne pepper, sea salt, and pepper. Pour the dressing over the kale mixture. For about one minute, gently massage oil mixture into vegetables by squeezing the vegetables and then releasing them into the bowl. *You will get your hands oily, but enjoy the sensual experience!*

3. Refrigerate in a sealed glass container for at least 15 minutes (or up to three days) to chill. Save a serving for tomorrow.

MINI TURKEY MEATBALLS

■ **MAKES ABOUT 12 MEATBALLS.**

I created this recipe while experimenting in the kitchen one day. Now I often make it on Sunday night, then use the meatballs for meals and snacks throughout the week.

Extra virgin olive oil cooking spray (I like Spectrum)
1 pound ground organic turkey meat
1 tablespoon ground flaxseeds
1 slice fresh Ezekiel bread (an organic sprouted whole-grain flourless bread), crusts removed, pulsed into crumbs in a food processor
¼ cup grated Parmesan cheese
⅓ cup finely shredded carrot
⅓ cup finely chopped white onion
2 large cloves garlic, finely diced (or ½ teaspoon garlic powder)
2 tablespoons minced fresh oregano leaves (or 1 tablespoon dried)
2 teaspoons minced fresh basil leaves (or 1 teaspoon dried)
1 organic egg, lightly beaten
½ teaspoon salt
Freshly ground black pepper and sea salt to taste

Preheat the broiler and spray a cookie sheet with cooking spray. Blend the turkey with all other ingredients in a large mixing bowl.

Shape into 1½-inch balls and place on the cookie sheet. Broil for 10 to 12 minutes, or until browned and cooked through.

Afternoon Snack

▶ ¼ cup all-natural organic hummus and sliced green peppers and carrots, or one serving of whole-grain crackers (I like Mary's Gone Crackers—all grain and no gluten)

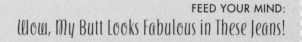

FEED YOUR MIND:

Wow, My Butt Looks Fabulous in These Jeans!

WRITE YOURSELF A nice note today, and post it on your bathroom mirror. Say something that will feed your heart, such as, "You are beautiful," "You rock," or "Stick with it; you can do it!"

Dinner

▶ Pork Tenderloin with Apple Chutney*
▶ Butternut Squash Quinoa*

I loved filming a Real Moms Love to Eat Chef Series event at Whole Foods Market in Chicago with executive chef team Brittany Ferrin and Vaidotas Karsokas of the Truffleberry Market in Westmont, Illinois. They're geniuses in the kitchen, and so easy to work with! Here is the entire delicious meal we created together—so healthy, you can lick the plate, guilt-free. The trick to making this meal is preparation ahead of time. Chop, roast, and marinate the day before and then "pull it all together" in thirty minutes the night you serve it!

SAGE PESTO

1 package (about 2 ounces) fresh sage
1 bunch (about 2 ounces) fresh basil
1 clove garlic
½ cup pine nuts or walnuts
3 tablespoons olive oil
1 tablespoon fresh lemon juice
½ cup freshly grated Parmesan cheese
Kosher salt and pepper to taste

In a blender or food processor, combine sage, basil, garlic, nuts, and oil. Blend until smooth. Stir in lemon, Parmesan, and salt and pepper to taste. Place in airtight container and chill, or pesto will turn brown.

PORK TENDERLOIN

■ **SERVES 4.**

1 pork tenderloin (about 1–1.5 lbs.)

1. Marinate pork overnight in *half* of the sage pesto, wrapped well. Save the other half of pesto for the cooked pork tenderloin.

2. Preheat oven to 375 degrees. Heat a large sauté pan with vegetable oil. Season the pork very well with kosher salt and fresh ground black pepper. Sear the pork all around in a very hot pan. Place in oven for 10 to 15 minutes or until a meat thermometer inserted into the middle reads 145 degrees. Pull the pork out of the oven and place on a resting rack. Rub the pork with the remaining pesto.

3. Let it rest for 10 to 15 minutes loosely covered with foil. Cut meat on a slightly angled bias and serve!

APPLE CHUTNEY

1 tablespoon butter
2 cups chopped yellow onion
½ teaspoon whole cloves
¼ teaspoon ground cinnamon
⅛ teaspoon ground cardamom
½ cup dried cranberries or cherries
½ cup packed brown sugar
¼ cup apple cider vinegar
5 cups chopped Gala apple
2 tablespoons chopped parsley (added after chutney is cooked)

Heat butter in a large saucepan or soup pot. Add all ingredients except apples; sauté about 5 minutes. Add apples. Cook about 15 minutes, stirring frequently. Discard cloves. Chill for later use or serve warm. Store leftovers in an airtight container in the refrigerator for up to two weeks.

BUTTERNUT SQUASH QUINOA

2 cups vegetable or chicken stock
2 cups dry quinoa, rinsed and drained
2 tablespoons olive oil
2 tablespoons champagne or white wine vinegar
1 clove garlic, finely chopped
1 roasted butternut squash, diced small
1 cup pine nuts, lightly toasted
¼ cup chopped parsley
Sea salt, to taste
Fresh ground black pepper, to taste
1 tablespoon chopped fresh oregano
1 tablespoon chopped fresh rosemary

1. Place the stock in a pot and bring it to a boil. Add the quinoa and cook until the liquid has absorbed and the quinoa is tender, about 10 minutes.

2. In a large bowl, stir together the rest of ingredients, except for the oregano and rosemary. Add a dash of salt and pepper, to taste.

3. Add the cooked quinoa to the bowl of ingredients and gently mix. Finish with the chopped herbs. Serve immediately.

NOTE: Tonight, skip ahead to tomorrow's menu and make the Raw Oatmeal, so it can soak overnight. See day four's midmorning snack.

DAY FOUR

Once a week, I like to have a totally raw day. This is that day! Try it—you'll feel fresh and rejuvenated.

Breakfast

▶ Green Smoothie (recipe from day one, with any additions you like)

▶ Fresh-cut fruit equivalent to one whole piece of fruit (cutting up fruit into a nice neat fruit salad is so appealing and elegant—fruit with a fork!)

Midmorning Snack

▶ Raw Oatmeal*

▶ 1 cup mixed berries

RAW OATMEAL

The night before, combine ¼ cup steel-cut oats and just enough filtered water to cover in a small covered glass container. Let it soak overnight in the refrigerator. By midmorning, the oats will be softened and ready to eat, right from the soaking container. I like to top them with just a pinch of stevia (this natural sweetener is very strong, so just a tiny pinch!), a dash of cinnamon, and 1 tablespoon raisins. Mix and enjoy.

FEED YOUR RELATIONSHIPS:
Cell Phones Aren't Just for Work!

CALL YOUR PARENTS or a special relative just to say hello and see how they are doing today.

Lunch

▶ Raw Nut Pâté (recipe on page 91)
▶ Savory Pizza Flax Crackers (recipe on page 96)
▶ Small side of leftover Energy Kale Salad from yesterday

Afternoon Snack

▶ Carrot-a-Mango Salad*

CARROT-A-MANGO SALAD

■ SERVES 4.

I love this salad recipe from my longtime dear friend Caren Yusem because of the flavor combination and radiant colors. It's so much like her, vibrant and beautiful.

4 carrots, grated
1 small ripe mango, peeled and thinly sliced
½ cup goat cheese crumbles
4 tablespoons of Orange Nut Dressing*
1½ tablespoons finely sliced scallions
1 teaspoon of finely chopped walnuts

Combine carrots, mango, and goat cheese crumbles in a glass bowl and toss well with dressing to evenly coat the salad; sprinkle with scallions and nuts, and enjoy immediately.

ORANGE SESAME DRESSING

■ SERVES 4.

4 tablespoons of orange juice
2 tablespoons of lemon juice
1 teaspoon of sesame oil
1 teaspoon of olive oil

Whisk all ingredients together and drizzle over greens or Carrot-a-Mango Salad.

FEED YOUR BODY:
Let's Play Footsie!

MAKE CIRCLES CLOCKWISE with your right foot twenty times, then your left foot, and reverse.

Dinner

▶ Sexy Raw Lasagna (see recipe on page 92—and save leftovers for two additional meals this week)

Optional: Dessert or Evening Snack

▶ Raw Brownies (see recipe on page 75)

DAY FIVE

Today is the day to "recycle" all those enticing leftovers, the fruits of your hard cooking labor all week—hooray, hooray, it's leftover day! And if you started this plan on a Monday, then bingo—it's Friday, the day to kick back. Lucky you!

Breakfast

▶ ChefMD's Warm and Nutty Cinnamon Quinoa*
▶ Leftover cut fruit

CHEFMD'S WARM AND NUTTY CINNAMON QUINOA

■ SERVES 4.

John La Puma, MD, a practicing physician and professionally trained chef in Santa Barbara, California, has been a guest on my radio show a couple of times, and each time, I learn something new and interesting. Check out his Web sites to learn more about this fantastic author of *ChefMD's Big Book of Culinary Medicine* (www://drjohnlapuma.com and http://ChefMD.com).

A few notes and tips from the book: low-fat soy or almond milk may replace the low-fat milk, blueberries may replace the blackberries, dark honey may replace the agave nectar, and walnuts may replace the pecans.

1 cup organic quinoa
1 cup organic 1% low-fat milk
1 cup water
2 cups fresh blackberries, organic preferred
½ teaspoon ground cinnamon
⅓ cup chopped pecans, toasted
4 teaspoons organic agave nectar (such as Madhava brand)

1. Rinse quinoa in a fine-mesh strainer; shake to remove excess water. Combine milk, water, and quinoa in a medium saucepan. Bring to a boil over high heat. Reduce heat to medium-low; cover and simmer 15 minutes or until most of the liquid is absorbed. Turn off heat; let stand covered 5 minutes.

2. While the quinoa cooks, roast the pecans in a 350-degree toaster oven for 5 to 6 minutes or in a dry skillet over medium heat for about 3 minutes.

3. Stir in blackberries and cinnamon; transfer to four bowls and top with pecans. Drizzle 1 teaspoon agave nectar over each serving.

Reprinted from the book *ChefMD's Big Book of Culinary Medicine* by John La Puma, MD, and Rebecca Powell Marx. Copyright ©

Midmorning Snack

► ½ cup low-fat cottage cheese mixed with chopped fresh fruit equaling one whole piece of fruit. This is one of my favorites from when I was in college.

► Or try this snack: My mother-in-law loves the creamy taste of low-fat cream cheese. For a nice midmorning snack, she'll put a little bit of cream cheese in an oven-proof container and warm it up just a little bit in her toaster oven. Then she'll add a few chopped green olives and eat it with baby carrots. Hits the spot!

► Or try a Green Smoothie with pineapple and a 1-inch square of leftover Raw Brownies (or are they all gone already?).

FEED YOUR MIND:
You Deserve It!

ARE YOU LIVING the life you want? What can you do to tweak things for the better? Devote two solid minutes to this thought: *I can live the life I want to live.*

Lunch

► Zone Diet Home-style Beef Vegetable Soup*

► Arugula Salad*

► 2 leftover Raw Brownies

ZONE DIET HOME-STYLE BEEF VEGETABLE SOUP

■ **SERVES 3 TO 4.**

Dr. Barry Sears is an international expert on hormonal responses induced by diet. He is the author of the number one *New York Times* bestseller *The Zone* and eleven other books on anti-inflammatory nutrition. Every time he is a guest on my radio show, I learn something new. Dr. Sears is such a wonderful man who has dedicated his life to helping others live healthier lives. He sent me this recipe from *Mastering the Zone* and says it's a mainstay to many Zoners. And by the way, "hiding" vegetables in soups is the best way to get kids to eat them. Refrigerate or freeze leftovers, then reheat for a quick meal or snack.

12 ounces lean ground beef (10 percent fat or less)
2½ cups diced celery
1 cup diced carrots
2 cups diced onions
2½ cups chopped tomatoes
½ cup tomato puree
2⅔ teaspoons olive oil
3 cups beef stock
Salt and pepper to taste
2 garlic cloves, minced, or to taste
⅛ teaspoon marjoram
⅛ teaspoon Worcestershire sauce
¼ teaspoon chives
1 teaspoon parsley
⅛ teaspoon oregano

Combine all the ingredients in a large saucepan. Bring to a boil; then simmer for 35 to 40 minutes, stirring occasionally, until all vegetables are tender.

ARUGULA SALAD

■ **SERVES 4.**

4 cups young arugula leaves, rinsed and dried
3 roma tomatoes, cut in quarters
¼ cup pine nuts
2 tablespoons olive oil
1 tablespoon fresh-squeezed lemon juice
¼ cup grated Parmesan cheese
Sea salt to taste
Freshly ground black pepper to taste.

Combine arugula, tomatoes, and pine nuts in a salad bowl. Whisk olive oil, lemon juice, cheese, sea salt, and pepper together. Toss dressing with salad mixture to coat.

Afternoon Snack

► Two or three more of those yummy Mini Meatballs
► Polish off the rest of that Energy Kale Salad

FEED YOUR BODY:
Rev It Up!

DO TWENTY JUMPING jacks! C'mon, you remember how. Nobody's watching. You'll get an instant energy boost.

Dinner

► Beth's Gor-met Ginger Chicken*
► ½ cup steamed rice

► One or two cups broccoli and cauliflower, mixed, or
any leftover raw vegetables from earlier in the week,
lightly steamed

BETH'S GOR-MET GINGER CHICKEN

■ **SERVES 4 TO 6.**

My family absolutely loves this chicken recipe, which is
music to a Real Mom's ears! This recipe tastes like something you'd get in a gourmet restaurant, but it's easy
enough to make at home.

Below my recipe, I've offered another more adult version, from Jenniffer Weigel, a columnist with the *Chicago
Tribune*, and author of two books, *Stay Tuned* and *I'm Spiritual, Dammit!* Her recipe is a more sophisticated version of
mine. Ginger and garlic are so healthy and are two of her
favorite flavors. Give it a whirl, but reserve it just for a special adult-only dinner, as all of the alcohol may not cook
off. It's your choice—both are delicious!

2 to 3 tablespoons of organic olive oil
1 to 2 pounds of boneless, skinless organic chicken breasts,
    cleaned and cut in strips
Dash or two of organic soy sauce (more or less, depending on
    taste)
Pinch of powdered organic ginger (more or less, depending on
    taste)
2 teaspoons of crumbled dried organic rosemary

1. Coat a large skillet with the oil. Add the chicken and soy sauce
and turn the chicken a few times using tongs, to coat it with oil.
Place the skillet over medium heat. Sprinkle the chicken with half
the powdered ginger and rosemary. Cook until about half cooked
through (5 minutes or so).

2. Using your tongs (wash them first, since they touched raw
chicken), turn the chicken pieces over and sprinkle with the remain-

ing ginger and rosemary. Cook until done, adding a little bit more oil and/or soy sauce if the pan gets too dry. Turn the pieces a few more times to make sure they are evenly golden brown, but do not overcook. You don't want dry chicken!

3. Serve over steamed rice, drizzled with any remaining sauce left in the pan after you remove the chicken.

JEN'S UNCLE RON'S GINGER CHICKEN

■ **SERVES 4.**

Here is Jenniffer Weigel's all-grown-up version. It actually comes from her uncle Ron's recipe.

Fresh gingerroot, about the size of 2 adult fingers—grated
3 cloves fresh garlic, smashed or very finely chopped
½ cup sherry or tawny port, drinking quality, not cooking type
⅓ cup fresh olive oil
4 tablespoons soy sauce
2 tablespoons sesame oil
3 tablespoons brown sugar
1½ pounds boneless, organic breast and thigh chicken meat

Place all ingredients into a large covered glass container and marinate 3 to 5 hours or overnight in the refrigerator. Grill the chicken and serve warm.

Optional Dessert

▶ Leftover Raw Brownie. Or wait until you get that late-night hunger attack, and polish off the Raw Lasagna!

DAY SIX

How are you doing? Loving food even more than you did before?
I hope so! Prepare for another delicious day.

Breakfast

▸ Banana smoothie: 1 banana (frozen or not—don't let
the lack of a frozen banana stop you from making a
smoothie!), 1 cup soy or rice milk, dash of vanilla extract, 1 tablespoon ground flaxseeds, 1 tablespoon
chocolate whey protein powder, and 1 tablespoon peanut butter

▸ Stonyfield Farm organic fat-free yogurt, any flavor

Midmorning Snack

▸ 4 pitted dates with a pecan or whole almond slipped
inside where the pit used to be (tastes just like pecan
pie—no kidding!) or ZonePerfect nutrition bar

▸ Apple or pear

FEED YOUR MIND:
Mini Meditation

FOCUS ON AN object for five minutes, like a ball or tree. It should
be something without any negative associations in your thoughts.
Visualize it in your mind, discovering the various details. Try to think
of nothing but the object. Let it consume your entire attention. It's
just five minutes; you can do it!

► 1 cup quinoa salad mixed with Lunchtime Qwik Chicken*

CHICKEN TIP:
Eliminate the Yuck Factor!

A HANDY TIP: Ask your butcher to cut up the boneless, skinless chicken breasts in the store for you, so when you get home, you don't have to cut or clean it—simply rinse and cook.

QUINOA SALAD

■ SERVES 3.

Cook quinoa just like you would cook rice; then fluff it with a fork and add a small handful (about ¼ cup) of pumpkin or sunflower seeds, a chopped carrot or other root vegetable, and a sprinkle of fresh parsley or cilantro if you have some around. Dress one cup cooled quinoa with 1 tablespoon olive oil, 1 tablespoon vinegar, and a dash of salt and pepper to taste. Don't be married to these directions, though—sometimes the best-tasting meals come when you improvise.

LUNCHTIME QWIK CHICKEN

1. Place 1 to 4 boneless skinless chicken breasts, sliced, in a pan over medium heat. Sauté with a sprinkle each of fresh rosemary, garlic powder (to taste), and two tablespoons of filtered water. Cook chicken through (about six minutes on each side) until golden brown. (Make more than you need—you'll be eating the leftovers tomorrow.)

2. Dice the cooked chicken and eat over the Quinoa Salad, above.

- ► Paper-thin Crisp Kale Chips*
- ► ½ cup pumpkin seeds, roasted and salted

FEED YOUR BODY:

Open Those Hips!

SEATED IN A chair, raise your right foot and rest your right ankle on your left knee. Oh, so gently, press down on your knee to open and stretch your hips. Repeat on the reverse side. This is great if you spend a lot of time sitting or standing.

PAPER-THIN CRISP KALE CHIPS

■ **SERVES 4 TO 6.**

Sometimes I like to bring these with me to the movie theater—they make the perfect snack!

1 tablespoon organic honey
1 tablespoon olive oil
1 teaspoon fresh-squeezed lime juice
One bag or bunch lacinato (dinosaur) kale
Pinch of sea salt

1. Line a baking sheet with a silicone liner (like Silpat) or waxed paper. In a bowl, combine honey, olive oil, and lime juice. Set aside.

2. Rinse the kale under cool water and salad-spin-dry thoroughly. If the kale is not completely dry, the kale chips will not cook; they will steam. So spin-dry it a second time. Anyone for a third round?

3. Rip the kale leaves into bite-size pieces, discarding the tough stems. Place them in a single layer on the silicone baking sheet and lightly sprinkle them with the honey mixture. Dehydrate at 120

degrees for approximately 8 hours. If you don't have a dehydrator, make these chips in your convection or regular oven at 350. Cook for 12 to 18 minutes.

4. For either cooking method, check to see whether the chips are done by gently touching them. If they are paper-thin and crackly, they're done. If soft and pliable, cook a little longer. Avoid over-cooking chips. If they turn brown, they will taste bitter.

5. Sprinkle with sea salt immediately after removing pan from the oven. (If you salt the chips before putting them in the oven, it will bring out the moisture in the kale and lengthen cooking time.)

Dinner

▶ 3-ounce steak filet

▶ One roasted sweet potato (but make two, so you have one for tomorrow's snack)

▶ 2 cups mixed greens with Oldways Dressing*

Can you say, "Steak, please"? I can, and do, a couple of times a month. However, I always eat steak on the days I know I will eat early in the evening, and then I take a walk to help boost my digestion. If you're going to eat meat, please eat the cleanest, leanest option available. Choose organic, free-range meat from local farmers, and always choose grass-fed beef. Simply cook steak to your preferred temperature in the broiler or on the grill with a light sprinkle of sea salt and Herbamare or Mrs. Dash seasoning.

To prepare the sweet potatoes, just roast in the oven for about one hour at 350 degrees. I like to put one teaspoon of coconut oil inside a slit on top of the potato while it cooks—the salty-sweet taste is delicious.

OLDWAYS DRESSING

■ **MAKES ABOUT 1 CUP**

> Georgia Orcutt, program manager at Oldways, a
> Mediterranean-lifestyle preservation organization, contrib-
> uted this recipe handed down by International Olive Oil
> Council executive director Fausto Luchetti and his wife,
> Mary. This special dressing will liven up any salad!

1 tablespoon sea salt
3 cloves garlic, minced
½ cup freshly squeezed lemon juice
½ cup high-quality extra virgin olive oil
Finely grated zest of 1 lemon

Mix together salt and minced garlic. In a jar with a lid, mix together lemon juice and olive oil. Add the salt and garlic mixture to
the lemon juice and olive oil, close the jar, and shake until well
combined. Serve over salad greens. Sprinkle the zest on top of the
salad just before serving.

Optional Dessert

► Tasty Chilly Lemon-shew Cookies*

TASTY CHILLY LEMON-SHEW COOKIES

> My rawsome-ly delightful friend Susie Sondag loves to
> make her lemon cookie recipe when friends come by. It's
> unbelievably easy to have these cookies on hand twenty-
> four/seven. I briefly mentioned how to make these in chap-
> ter five, but here is a slightly fancier version.

1 cup soaked cashews (soak in water in glass jar in refrigerator
   overnight)
2 tablespoons agave nectar or honey
1½ tablespoons lemon juice
1 tablespoon plus 1 teaspoon lemon zest, finely chopped
½ teaspoon vanilla
⅛ teaspoon sea salt

Blend all the ingredients together in the Vitamix, blender, or food
processor until the mixture turns into dough. Roll out and use a
round cookie cutter to make cookies and place in freezer to nibble
on anytime!

DAY SEVEN

*This is the last day I'll make a day-by-day note for you—I think
you're doing a great job; you're on track, and you're rocking it. So
just keep going, Real Mom! You're heading in a great direction.*

Breakfast

▶ Spinnie Scramble: Scramble two eggs with about ½
  cup lightly steamed spinach and half a chopped onion.
  Season with sea salt and cracked black pepper.

▶ 1 small patty apple-flavored chicken sausage: Sauté
  patty with a few drops of olive oil.

Midmorning Snack

▶ 10 frozen grapes (I always keep a stash in the freezer—
  like mini Popsicle bites!)

▶ 1 small round of Babybel cheese (individually wrapped
  in wax disks)

▶ Handful of roasted walnuts and almonds (with or
  without salt)

Empty the Bucket!

CLEAR YOUR MIND. Wipe the slate clean of all the internal chatter. If you think of something, acknowledge it and set it free, like a balloon in the wind. See if you can keep your mind totally still and empty for one full minute. It's harder than you think, but the more you practice, the more you will flex your mental muscle!

Lunch

- ► 2 cups Vegetarian Corn, Cashew, and Okra Gumbo*

- ► ½ cup cooked rice

- ► Salad of baby spring greens, sliced peaches, yellow peppers, and orange cherry tomatoes tossed with Balsamic Vinaigrette* and a few slices of Lunchtime Qwik Chicken left over from yesterday

BALSAMIC VINAIGRETTE

■ **MAKES ABOUT 1 CUP.**

¾ cup olive oil
¼ cup balsamic vinegar
1 dash of stevia sweetener
½ teaspoon garlic powder or 1 teaspoon minced garlic
½ teaspoon sea salt
½ teaspoon freshly ground black pepper

Whisk all ingredients together and drizzle over fresh greens or any salad.

VEGETARIAN CORN, CASHEW, AND OKRA GUMBO

■ **MAKES ABOUT 4 SERVINGS.**

This recipe takes some effort, but it's so worthwhile. Emmy Award–winning documentary filmmaker Gaylon Emerzian's passion for food led her to found the James Beard Award–winning Web site www.Spatulatta.com. Gaylon is also a cookbook writer and coproducer of the Beard-nominated *Living on the Wedge: Wisconsin's Artisan Cheesemakers*, an hour-long documentary for Wisconsin Public Broadcasting. This is her recipe.

2 ears of corn on the cob, in their husks
1 cup vegetable oil
1 cup flour
3 stalks celery, coarsely chopped
1 large onion, coarsely chopped
1 large green pepper, coarsely chopped
3 cloves garlic, finely chopped
3 cups vegetable broth
1 16-ounce can tomatoes
1½ tablespoons chopped fresh thyme
1 tablespoon serrano or habanero pepper, finely chopped (optional)
1½ cups okra, cut into chunks
2 tablespoons Spice House smoked paprika (or use any paprika)
1 cup raw cashews

1. Roast the corn on the cob ahead of time: Soak the ears of corn with the husks on in water for 30 minutes. Put them on the grill, turning as the husks begin to burn. You want some of the kernels to darken on the edges but not burn. Cool, cut the kernels off the cob, and set them aside. This can be done days ahead of time if you freeze the kernels.

2. Next, make a roux. Combine the oil and flour in a heavy (preferably cast-iron) pan and stir constantly over medium heat until the roux is a dark reddish brown color. [Note from me: This could take

a very long time—up to an hour or more! You may need to stir a bit, do something else, come back, stir a bit, etc. Just keep an eye on it so it doesn't burn, and be patient—the mind-blowing taste will be worth it!] Alternatively, you can make roux in the microwave: Place the oil and flour in a large glass measuring cup. Cook on high for 6 minutes. Whisk out the lumps and cook for another 3 minutes. Whisk again and check color. Be aware that the mixture will be extremely hot and will continue to cook even after it is removed from the microwave. Stir it to distribute the heat (and color) from the core. When the roux has reached the correct color, pour it into a big soup pot or Dutch oven and put it over medium heat.

3. Add the Creole "holy trinity" to the roux—the celery, onion, and green pepper. Sauté it for a few minutes until coated. Add the garlic and sauté for 1 minute more. Add the broth, tomatoes, thyme, hot pepper, and corn. Simmer for 40 minutes.

4. Add the okra and the paprika. Simmer for 15 more minutes. Adding the okra near the finish keeps it from breaking down.

5. Add the cashews last and cook for 5 to 7 minutes, just until they are heated through. Cooking too long will make the nuts fall apart.

6. Serve with or over cooked brown or white rice.

Afternoon Snack

▶ Leftover Quinoa Salad with Lunchtime Qwik Chicken (use about ½ cup) rolled in a Rudi's Organic Bakery 7 Grain with Flax wrap

FEED YOUR HEART:
Speak of Love!

WHOM DO YOU love? Have you told them lately? No? Well, then, what are you waiting for? You must tell them *immediately*! Do it now. It's more important than that other thing you were about to do.

- 1 cup pasta with Sleep-deprived Alfredo Sauce* or rice
- Cocoon Chicken*
- 1 cup (or more) any steamed veggies drizzled with olive oil and sprinkled with sea salt

SUPER EASY NO-BRAIN-NECESSARY SLEEP-DEPRIVED ALFREDO SAUCE

My busy friend Tanya Bennett is a mother of two, writer, and musician who is on a quest to enjoy more quality time. She came up with this recipe one sleep-deprived hungry evening—it's perfect topped with the Cocoon Chicken, recipe below.

This is barely even a recipe. Just cook the amount of pasta you want to make (about 2 ounces per person), drain it, put it back on the stove, add about 1 tablespoon butter per serving and a dollop (more or less) of organic low-fat sour cream. Sprinkle with your desired amount of grated Parmesan cheese, sea salt, and pepper. Talk about easy! You could make this in your sleep.

COCOON CHICKEN

Busy with kids' after-school activities? Here's the perfect dinner, courtesy of one of my longtime close friends, Wini Nimrod. It's the perfect meat addition to any salad or meal. It's barely a recipe either. Just take a frozen chicken breast, smear it with coconut oil or olive oil, sprinkle with your favorite seasoning (like Herbamare or Mrs. Dash) and a little sea salt, wrap it in foil (that's the cocoon part), and bake it in the oven at 375 degrees for about 20 minutes.

Sometimes I call this "Multitasking Chicken," because while the chicken is cooking, we Real Moms can check our e-mails and fold

some laundry while the kids do their homework at the kitchen table (in anticipation of the dinner to come).

You could also serve this with steamed rice instead of the pasta and Alfredo, depending on what sounds good to you this evening. Top the rice with a dash of soy sauce and a dab of butter (in my book, one dab = 1 teaspoon). Or stir-fry it with some olive oil and slivered green onions, a nice quick way to boost the flavor of plain rice when you have the time.

DAY EIGHT

Breakfast

- ▶ Green Smoothie (all fruit, skipping the nut butter today)
- ▶ 1 or 2 hard-boiled eggs, sliced, with sea salt sprinkled on top

Midmorning Snack

- ▶ Chocolate smoothie (make this one with 1 banana, 1 cup soy or rice milk, a dash of vanilla extract, 1 tablespoon ground flaxseed, and 1 tablespoon raw cacao powder. Blend and enjoy—and don't let anyone tell you that you can't have two smoothies in one day!)
- ▶ 15 to 20 roasted almonds (salted or not)

Lunch

- ▶ Easy, Foolproof Lentil and Barley Soup*

EASY, FOOLPROOF LENTIL AND BARLEY SOUP

■ **SERVES AT LEAST 6.**

My friend Jane Bernstein shares this recipe with us from her grandmother.

1 cup lentils
1½ quarts (6 cups) water
½ cup barley
1 onion, chopped
2 celery stalks, chopped
1 carrot, chopped
1 potato, diced
1 16-ounce can tomatoes
1½ teaspoons salt
⅛ teaspoon black pepper
1 clove garlic, minced
1 handful fresh parsley, minced

In a big soup pot, combine all ingredients and bring to a boil. Reduce the heat and simmer, covered, for an hour, stirring occasionally. Just before serving, mince a handful of fresh parsley and stir it into the pot. This soup is great as soon as it's ready, and delicious for the next few days. Add hot sauce to taste. This recipe doubles nicely for a huge pot of hearty soup.

Afternoon Snack

- ▶ 1 to 2 ounces of Whole Foods Market 365 Organic turkey jerky (or you can find your favorite brand at any natural grocery store)

- ▶ Small piece of sliced fruit, like kiwi or pears

FEED YOUR BODY:
Drum Majorette March!

MARCH IN PLACE for a count of fifty, knees high, swinging your arms. Feel your heart pump. Really give it all you've got—do it up so big that it would absolutely *humiliate* your kids if they saw you. (Resist the urge to repeat when you pick them up from school.)

Dinner

- ▶ Savory Avocado Soup*

SAVORY AVOCADO SOUP

■ SERVES 4 TO 6.

This recipe comes from Bernadette Penotti, a celebrated health and fitness consultant and sought-after intuitive self-care strategist.

3 to 5 ripe plum tomatoes or 1 basket cherry tomatoes
½ cup sun-dried tomatoes
1 ripe avocado, peeled and pitted
2 to 3 large handfuls of spinach
A few sprigs of basil (stems removed)
5 to 6 pitted black olives
½ red bell pepper, cored and seeded

1 stalk celery
dash of cayenne pepper (optional)

1. In the bowl of your blender or Vitamix, add all but ½ cup of tomatoes (chopped). Blend for a few pulses until smooth. Add the avocados, spinach, and basil, and blend a few pulses after each.

2. Chop the olives and bell pepper. Stir into the soup along with the remaining tomatoes. Add optional cayenne pepper if you like it spicy. (I might also add a little minced garlic and maybe a pinch of sea salt, but that's just me. You can also experiment with other veggies, like baby carrots, cucumbers, scallions, or other herbs, like dill and cilantro. You could garnish this soup with raw nori [a sea vegetable] or crumbled raw flax crackers for a sublime, supereasy, nutritious meal on the go!)

3. Ladle into bowls or mugs; then serve.

When I enjoy a delicious bowl of soup for a light dinner, I always add a side of sliced chicken breast for protein. I love the Bell & Evans precooked frozen chicken breasts. I simply heat one up in the toaster oven at 350 degrees with a teaspoon of olive oil and some sea salt sprinkled on top. By the time I ladle out the soup, my chicken is heated and ready to slice. I serve it on a small salad plate with a nice little lettuce garnish or sliced carrots for appeal. Simple, delicious, and healthy.

KITCHEN TIP:
The Many Faces of Garbanzo Beans

MY GOOD FRIEND Teri Knapp, TV producer, wife, and Real Mom to two teens, loves garbanzo beans. The real thing. The canned ones taste like paste to her (me too) and will ruin a dish. Instead, she soaks a bag of dried beans in a bowl overnight, then gives them a rinse in the morning and boils them until soft. (You can also cook

(continued)

them in your slow cooker.) Then she'll use them in various ways throughout the week: added to tabouleh, in place of croutons in a salad, as a protein to replace a meat portion, or just on their own with a little salad dressing. You can also let them dry really well on a kitchen towel, then sauté them until they get crisp and golden brown. Put them out in a bowl instead of nuts at cocktail hour—they'll be a hit! Thanks for the hint, Teri.

Optional Dessert

▶ Citrus Almond Cake*

CITRUS ALMOND CAKE

■ SERVES 6 TO 8.

This flavorful and festive cake comes from my friend Sharon Meyers. She first learned to make it when she lived in the Middle East. It offers the tang of both lemon and orange, and the added interest of cardamom, without any flour! It's a great dessert for people who avoid wheat or gluten. Warning: This is hardly a low-calorie dessert. You'll understand what I mean when you taste it. Keep your portion small—about a half-inch slice should be just about right for a decadent taste and pleasure without the guilt.

2 organic oranges
2 organic lemons
6 organic eggs
1 cup organic light brown sugar, packed
2 cups organic almonds, finely ground (you can do this yourself with a Vitamix blender/food processor)
1 teaspoon each baking powder and cardamom
Powdered sugar for garnish

1. Place whole lemons and oranges into a small pot in enough water to cover them, and bring to a boil. Simmer, covered, for one hour.

2. Preheat the oven to 350 degrees. Drain and cut each citrus fruit in half, discarding seeds. Process in a blender or food processor until smooth. Put in bowl and set aside.

3. Beat the eggs and sugar together until well blended, then add the fruit puree, almonds, baking powder, and cardamom. Stir just until blended.

4. Pour the batter into a lightly oiled springform pan and bake for one hour, or until the top feels firm to the touch.

5. Cool, then cut into slices and serve with a dusting of powdered sugar.

DAY NINE

Breakfast

► Green Smoothie with 1 tablespoon nut butter and 1 tablespoon raw cacao powder

► Kashi GOLEAN Crunch Honey Almond Flax cereal with rice milk

Midmorning Snack

► A handful of mixed sunflower seeds and nuts (or trail mix)

► ½ cup dried mango slices

► 1 cup cold Lifeway Kefir Chocolate Truffle drink (or chocolate soy or rice milk)

Lunch

► Easy Open-face Tacos*

EASY OPEN-FACE TACOS

■ **SERVES 4 TO 6.**

This tasty recipe comes from my friend and fellow nutrition aficionado Deborah Enos, known as the "One-Minute Wellness Coach," who helps us all get healthy in seconds.

1 pound organic ground beef
1 tablespoon olive oil
1 can (about 15 ounces) refried beans
1 can (about 15 ounces) black beans, rinsed and drained
½ container (about 8 ounces or 1 cup) salsa
1 cup beef broth
Juice from 1 lime
2 cups baked tortilla chips
4 cups chopped green salad
¼ cup grated cheese

1. Sauté beef in one tablespoon of olive oil for 5 minutes. Add the can of refried beans and the strained black beans. Combine and cook for 3 to 4 minutes. Add beef broth and salsa, and let simmer for 3 to 5 minutes. Add the lime juice.

2. Cover a platter with baked chips. Put the taco mixture onto the chips, then top with green salad, remaining salsa, and grated cheese. Serve with salad tongs—everyone can help themselves!

————

Afternoon Snack

► Hot Mom Sweet Potato Quesadilla*

HOT MOM SWEET POTATO QUESADILLA

Jessica Denay, my dear friend and founder of Hot Moms Club and author of the Hot Mom's Handbook series, says this is her go-to snack. Her son eats it too, hold the cilantro.
    This is a Hot Mom power snack if ever there was one! You can adjust the amounts according to how many you want to make—one just for you, or make them for the whole family for a quick meal.

Organic sweet potatoes (or butternut squash), about ½ potato
    per serving
Black beans (about ½ cup per serving)
Chopped cilantro, about 1 tablespoon per serving
Organic whole-wheat tortillas (2 per serving, about 6 inches in
    diameter)
Shredded sharp cheddar cheese, about 1 tablespoon per serving
Greek yogurt (instead of sour cream), about 1 tablespoon per
    serving (I like FAGE)

1. Bake the sweet potato (or squash) at about 350 degrees for up to an hour. Cool, peel, and cut into chunks (you can do this ahead of time and keep them in the refrigerator).

2. Heat the black beans; then add them to the sweet potato chunks. Stir in the cilantro. Heat a griddle or skillet over medium heat and place a tortilla on the hot surface. Scoop the sweet potato/bean mixture onto the warm tortilla. Sprinkle the cheese on top. Cover

REAL MOMS LOVE TO EAT

241

BETH ALDRICH

with a second tortilla. Peek under the quesadilla to see if it is browned yet. When it looks crisp and golden, flip it over carefully. When both sides are done, remove it to a plate, cut into fourths, and serve with the Greek yogurt.

FEED YOUR RELATIONSHIPS:

Your BFF!

DO YOU HAVE a best friend? What makes her special to you? Provide your dearest friend with a short list: "I hope you realize how important you are to me. These are just a few reasons why. . . ."

Dinner

► 2 slices Chica-boom Pizza*
► Goat Cheese and Pear Salad*

CHICA-BOOM PIZZA

■ SERVES 4.

When I first got married and was learning my way around the kitchen, I would make this pizza for my husband, switching it up with different toppings each time. This is easy because it uses prepared ingredients, but you can't tell from the taste. He fell in love all over again.

1 12-inch Rustic Crust Old World ready-to-bake pizza crust (I like the Organic Great Grains flavor, full of whole grains, including omega-3-rich flaxseeds)
1 cup of Amy's organic tomato-basil pasta sauce
1 cup diced cooked chicken breast (if you don't buy it precooked, sauté in olive oil, garlic, and rosemary and then cut into pieces)

1 cup of diced and sliced veggies of your choice—the more the
merrier
1 cup of Organic Valley Family of Farms shredded mozzarella
cheese

Preheat the oven to 450 degrees. Spread a thin layer of tomato sauce
on top of pizza crust, arrange chicken and vegetables on top of
sauce, sprinkle cheese on top, covering all the ingredients, and bake
for 8 to 12 minutes or until cheese begins to bubble and get a bit
brown on the outside edges of the pizza. Let sit for a few minutes
to cool and to set the cheese. Slice and enjoy!

GOAT CHEESE AND PEAR SALAD

■ SERVES 1.

My sister-in-law from New York always has the best salad
recipes. When she pulled this one together for me, I immediately thought of you! So here it is. This makes one plate,
but you can make as many plates as you want, of course.
Just increase the ingredients accordingly.

Fresh Romaine lettuce
1 sliced Bosc pear
2 ounces goat cheese (crumbled—blocks and wedges crumble
better if you put them in the freezer for about 30 minutes)
2 slices cooked bacon, crumbled
A sprinkle of diced red onion
A few cherry tomatoes or chopped plum tomatoes
A sprinkle of freshly minced garlic

Arrange ingredients on a plate and serve with oil, vinegar, salt, and
pepper.

Breakfast

- ▶ 2 hard-boiled eggs seasoned with sea salt
- ▶ I Spy Waffle*

I SPY WAFFLES

I've been making this recipe for years (passed down in my family for generations). I added the flaxseeds, though—my twenty-first-century adaptation! Nobody ever notices them, but they do everyone good. (By the way, the first waffle never turns out as perfectly as the subsequent ones, so I always keep that one for myself and top with a dollop of pure maple syrup. We Real Moms are such martyrs!)

1½ cups whole-wheat or organic white flour
1 tablespoon ground flaxseeds (the secret ingredient!)
1½ teaspoons baking powder
⅛ teaspoon sea salt
1½ cups milk (I use rice milk)
2 eggs
3 tablespoons sunflower oil (or any light vegetable oil)
2 tablespoons agave nectar
Sliced strawberries and organic maple syrup for garnish

1. Preheat the waffle iron and spray lightly with cooking spray. Combine flour, flaxseed, baking powder, and sea salt in a bowl until blended and set aside. In a separate bowl, whisk together the milk, eggs, oil, and agave nectar.

2. Combine the dry and wet ingredients to make batter—stir just until blended. Pour about ½ cup of batter at a time onto the hot waffle iron and cook, turning once (I literally flip my iron over on the counter so the waffle cooks through properly, but if yours turns

out fine without doing that, then follow the instructions on your own iron).

3. Serve with sliced strawberries and maple syrup.

Midmorning Snack

▶ Green Smoothie (your choice of special ingredients!)

▶ ¼ cup mixed nuts

> FEED YOUR SPIRIT:
> ### Be a Tree Hugger!
>
> HAVE YOU EVER hugged a tree? No, seriously! Have you ever planted a tree, or even pressed the beautiful leaf of a tree in a book? If not, I highly recommend getting more closely acquainted with trees. You can feel their energy—they are one of the most primal and integral parts of our planet. They literally maintain our atmosphere. They allow us to live here. Give them some love!

Lunch

▶ Summer Sun Bean Dip*

SUMMER SUN BEAN DIP

■ **MAKES ENOUGH FOR 3 OR 4 FRIENDS TO SHARE.**

My dear friend and Real Mom Kristie, who lives next door to my summer cottage, loves to get together on the screened-in porch and share stories while we watch the children enjoying the free-and-easy days of summer on the shore. While we love our delicious meals and summer salads, this tasty bean dip really hits the spot on those beachy days when you just want to munch for lunch. It's really more of a salad than a bean dip, but it is pretty darned good with baked tortilla chips! Here's to sand in your shoes and bean dip on your plate! This recipe was handed down to her from her mother, who has been making it for years.

IMPORTANT NOTE: For this recipe, drain and rinse in a colander anything that comes out of a can to get rid of excess liquid and salt. Just drain the pimentos; no need to rinse those.

1. In a large bowl, mix the following together:

   1 or 2 15-ounce cans black-eyed peas
   1 15-ounce can pinto beans
   1 15-ounce can of black beans
   1 11-ounce can shoepeg (white) corn
   1 small jar diced pimento
   1 medium onion diced (white or red)
   1 cup chopped celery (about 2 stalks)
   1 cup chopped green pepper (about 1 large)
   2 peeled, seeded, finely chopped jalapeño peppers

2. Now make the marinade. In a saucepan, combine the following and bring them to a boil:

   1 teaspoon salt
   ½ teaspoon black pepper
   1 tablespoon water
   ¾ cup cider vinegar
   ½ cup vegetable oil
   1 cup sugar (can substitute agave nectar)

3. After the mixture is boiling, remove it from the heat and pour it over the bean mixture. Refrigerate and drain before serving. (Lucky for us summer Real Moms, this can be made the night before—it will taste even better the next day.)

4. Serve with carrots, celery, and/or a few organic corn chips.

Afternoon Snack

- ½ cup pumpkin seeds in the shell (they take longer to eat this way)

- 1 container Earthbound Farm organic prepackaged mini carrots and ranch dip

FEED YOUR BODY:
Roll with It

BUSY DAY? STOP the madness for a few seconds and do five very slow neck rolls in a clockwise direction, and five more in a counter-clockwise direction. There, now, doesn't that feel better?

Dinner

- Gwen's Shrimp Pasta in a Snap*

- Mixed green salad with a drizzle of your favorite dressing

GWEN'S SHRIMP PASTA IN A SNAP

■ SERVES 4.

Gwen Solberg, mother of two, was one of the original co-founders of Healthy Handfuls snacks for kids. When we met, we instantly became the best of friends, and our passion for healthy eating and finding happiness in every day has kept us close ever since.

8 ounces organic whole-wheat or low-carb pasta
4 cups sliced asparagus (cut into 1-inch pieces)
1 pound peeled and deveined shrimp, coarsely chopped
2 or 3 tablespoons organic olive oil, divided

1 cup fresh basil leaves
Juice from half a fresh lemon
2 garlic cloves, minced
A splash of water (maybe 2 tablespoons)
Sea salt, to taste

1. Cook the pasta according to the directions, drain, and set aside.

2. Heat a skillet over medium and add the asparagus, shrimp, and 1 tablespoon of the olive oil. Toss and combine, sautéing for about 5 minutes, until the shrimp turns white-pink, indicating it is cooked through. Remove from the heat and set aside.

3. In a Vitamix or blender, combine basil, lemon juice, garlic, water, the remaining olive oil, and salt. Blend on high until pureed and slightly heated up from the heat of the blender.

4. Divide pasta among four plates. Top each with one-fourth of the asparagus-shrimp mixture and drizzle one-fourth of the sauce over each plate. *Buon Appetito!*

Optional Dessert

▶ Simply Pretty Party Dessert: Sorbet Sundae*

SIMPLY PRETTY PARTY DESSERT: SORBET SUNDAE

■ SERVES 1.

My dear friend, Web site editor, and right-hand gal Daisy Simmons loves her simple sweet dessert contribution. I do too, so today we're having it as a special treat.

1 scoop raspberry sorbet
1 scoop mango sorbet
2 tablespoons vanilla soy yogurt
¾ tablespoon chopped almonds

3 to 5 blackberries
1 mint sprig

1. Scoop raspberry sorbet into a small tumbler, pressing down with a spoon to smooth. Add a tablespoon of yogurt, then sprinkle half the almonds on top.

2. Scoop your mango sorbet neatly on top, then repeat with the yogurt and nuts. Put the berries on top and garnish with mint. Chill until time to eat.

DAY ELEVEN

Breakfast

▶ Steel-cut oatmeal sprinkled with a little bit of stevia and cinnamon and topped with 1 sliced banana

▶ Hard-boiled egg, seasoned with sea salt

Midmorning Snack

▶ Gingered Pear Green Smoothie*

GINGERED PEAR GREEN SMOOTHIE

■ SERVES 2.

Here's another delish and healthy recipe from Bernadette Penotti.

2 pears, cored
1 whole lemon, peeled and seeded
1 cup water
½-inch nub of ginger, peeled

3 huge handfuls of kale, chard, or spinach (chopped and big
stems removed)

Blend everything together in the Vitamix or blender and savor!

FEED YOUR MIND:
Do It Write!

DO YOU WRITE in a journal or record your dreams each morning?
Writing helps clear your mind and clarify your thoughts, making
room for more creativity. It doesn't matter if your writing is "good."
It's just an exercise, for you and you alone.

Lunch

► Harvest Pumpkin and Black Bean Soup*

HARVEST PUMPKIN AND BLACK BEAN SOUP

■ SERVES ABOUT 8.

> I discovered this luscious recipe on Noel's Kitchen Tips
> blog and have been a fan ever since.

2 tablespoons butter
1 medium onion, diced
4 garlic cloves, pressed through a garlic press (or minced)
1 15-ounce can black beans, rinsed and drained
1 30-ounce can pumpkin puree
1 14.5-ounce can diced tomatoes with juice
1 teaspoon sugar
1 teaspoon cumin
1 teaspoon chili powder
1 teaspoon pepper

1 teaspoon Spanish paprika
4 cups beef broth
½ cup heavy cream
Chives, celery leaves, or croutons for garnish

1. In a stockpot, melt the butter and sauté onions and garlic until they are translucent. Add black beans, pumpkin puree, and tomatoes, stirring until combined. Add sugar, cumin, chili powder, pepper, paprika, beef broth, and cream. Simmer on low heat for 20 minutes. (This soup can be served as is, or pureed in a blender before serving.)

2. Ladle into bowls and garnish with chopped chives, celery leaves, or croutons.

Afternoon Snack

▶ 20 salted, roasted almonds or ThinkThin Mini Bite Bar

▶ One (you heard me, just one) ounce of delightful, rich, dark chocolate

I typically purchase a bar of Green & Black's or Vosges gourmet chocolate and break off one square as a midday treat. It's also an elegant dessert with sliced strawberries. For best results: nibble!

FEED YOUR PASSION:
O, Mighty Chocolate Gods . . .

GIVE THANKS TO the chocolate gods! It's not idolatry—it's *chocolate*! Aren't you glad you have it in your life?

- ▶ Flax-crusted Tilapia*
- ▶ Roasted Asparagus Tips*

FLAX-CRUSTED TILAPIA

■ **SERVES 4.**

4 tilapia fish fillets
1 lemon
1 tablespoon fresh or 1 teaspoon dried dill
1 tablespoon ground flaxseeds
1 teaspoon Herbamare (or other favorite) seasoning

Heat a skillet over medium-high heat. Spray with cooking spray. Sprinkle each fish fillet with the lemon, dill, flaxseeds, and seasoning. Put the fish in the hot pan and cook until golden brown. Flip and cook remaining side until the fish flakes with a fork.

ROASTED ASPARAGUS TIPS

■ **SERVES 4.**

20 asparagus spears
1 tablespoon olive oil
1 teaspoon sea salt

Preheat the oven to 450 degrees. Trim off tough bottoms of asparagus spears and arrange them in a shallow pan, about ¼ inch apart. Drizzle with olive oil and sprinkle with salt. Roast for about 8 minutes, or to desired tenderness. Serve hot.

NOTE: Set aside four spears of Roasted Asparagus Tips for tomorrow's snack!

Optional Dessert

- Luna & Larry's Coconut Bliss. This frozen nondairy, nonsoy "ice cream" is a super way to get some dessert lovin' through all-natural ingredients. They have a variety of yummy flavors.

DAY TWELVE

Breakfast

- Green Smoothie with frozen berries
- Slice of Ezekiel raisin toast with just a bit of organic butter

FEED YOUR SPIRIT:
I DO BELIEVE!

WHAT DO YOU believe in? Stand up for what matters to you! I believe in protecting the planet.

Midmorning Snack

- Slice of whole-grain toast with a thin spread of Nutella and thinly sliced banana

Lunch

- Spaghetti Primavera*

There are days when I just need pasta. Today's that day. I love Dreamfields pasta, which has five grams of fiber and only five digestible carbs per serving. Dreamfields pasta contributed this yummy recipe, which you may eat guilt-free. The veggies in this dish take the place of my salad for lunch.

SPAGHETTI PRIMAVERA

■ **SERVES 6.**

1 box Dreamfields spaghetti
2 tablespoons olive oil
2 small zucchini, shredded
2 medium carrots, peeled and shredded
1 large red bell pepper, cut into small thin strips
2 shallots, minced
⅓ cup grated Parmesan cheese
Salt and freshly ground black pepper

1. Cook pasta according to package directions. Meanwhile, heat oil in medium skillet over medium heat. Cook zucchini, carrots, bell pepper, and shallots 5 minutes, or until tender, stirring frequently.

2. Drain pasta. Add to skillet; toss with vegetable mixture, adding half of the cheese while tossing. Season with salt and pepper to taste. Serve with remaining cheese.

Afternoon Snack

▶ Leftover grilled asparagus tossed with a little bit of good olive oil and a sprinkle of feta cheese

---

FEED YOUR BODY:
Feeling Crunchy?

STOP, GET ON the floor, and do twenty-five crunches before your snack. I know you worked out this morning, but why not do more? It takes less than sixty seconds . . . feed your body!

Dinner

▶ Suz's Salad*

SUZ'S SALAD

■ SERVES 6.

> I love it when my sister-in-law makes this simply delicious
> salad for me when I visit.

12 cups spring salad greens mix
2 cups arugula
1 cup crumbled goat cheese
1 apple, sliced
½ cup dried cranberries
¼ cup sliced almonds or walnut pieces

Toss all ingredients together, then toss with an organic store-bought
Italian dressing or just ½ cup olive oil, juice from one lemon, and
salt and pepper to taste. If you have any leftover cooked meat, such
as chicken, shrimp, or steak, you could toss that in as well (this is a
good way to make use of restaurant leftovers).

DAY THIRTEEN

Breakfast

▶ Banana Smooshers*

▶ 2 soft-boiled eggs, sliced and topped with paprika and
sea salt

BANANA SMOOSHERS

One of my best friends, Wini Nimrod, loves to nibble on these snacks throughout the day. They're a great pick-me-up snack, but I also love them for breakfast!

Mash a ripe banana on rice cakes, crackers, or toast. Top with a sprinkle of cinnamon.

FEED YOUR MIND:
Puzzle It

KEEP YOUR MIND as sharp as a tack: spend 10 minutes doing a sudoku, crossword, or other puzzle.

Midmorning Snack

► Polenta*

POLENTA

Polenta (a.k.a. Italian grits) is made from coarsely ground cornmeal and is a staple of northern Italy. It can take on many flavors—what are you in the mood for?

Bring 1 cup of water and a dash of salt to a boil. Slowly add ⅓ cup polenta and stir (lower heat so it doesn't splash all over) for about 5 minutes. Instant comfort food! This is good with a savory or sweet topping, depending on what you're in the mood for—try a dash of olive oil, a sprinkle of garlic powder, some chopped fresh tomatoes, and a little dried oregano, or go sweet with a drizzle of maple syrup, a dab of butter, and a splash of milk.

▶ Double-duty Chicken Salad*

DOUBLE-DUTY CHICKEN SALAD

■ SERVES 4.

My sister-in-law Deanna makes this delish salad, then uses the rest of the chicken for a yummy soup. Save the soup for tomorrow. (It will taste even better by then anyway.)

8 boneless, skinless chicken breasts
⅓ cup light mayonnaise
1 cup chopped celery
½ cup finely chopped onion
1 apple, cored and coarsely chopped
Salt and pepper to taste

Boil the chicken breasts (reserve the liquid), cool, and dice. Put half the chicken aside for soup (see the following recipe). Put the other half in a bowl with the mayonnaise and stir to coat. Add celery, onion, and apple, and stir to combine. Add salt and pepper. Serve immediately, or refrigerate and serve chilled.

DOUBLE-DUTY SOUP

■ SERVES 8.

For this easy soup, just combine the leftover chicken from the Double-duty Chicken Salad in a saucepan or soup pot with 1 cup cooked brown rice or whole-grain pasta, 1 cup diced celery, 1 cup chopped onion, ½ cup chopped carrot, or any other vegetables you have in your crisper. Add 6 to 8 cups vegetable or chicken broth. Heat over medium heat until the vegetables are tender, about 30 minutes. Season with salt and pepper. Save this for lunch tomorrow.

Afternoon Snack

- ► 1 cup Miso Broth*
- ► Julienne-cut veggies, hummus, and roasted turkey breast wrapped in lettuce leaves

MISO BROTH

Put a heaping teaspoon of miso (a salty paste of cooked and aged soybeans) in a big tea mug, add almost boiling water, stir till the miso is dissolved, and enjoy. Warming and nourishing.

Dinner

- ► Power Rice and Beans*
- ► Chopped salad of romaine, mixed baby greens, yellow tomato, red pepper, carrots, and celery (or whatever fresh veggies you have)

Be a Soup-er Hostess!

MY TV PRODUCER friend and Real Mom Teri Knapp loves to give dinner parties, and she spends a lot of time planning and prepping for them. It makes her crazy that guests fill up on hors d'oeuvres while waiting for the main event, so she's done away with cheese platters and dips, and serves hot or cold soups instead. What a great idea! Creamy comfort soups in the fall and winter, cold and crisp soups in the warmer months (gazpacho is the most popular, and hot sauce is optional). Cold soups can be presented in a long-stemmed, big-bowled wineglass for sipping, and hot soups are served in a mug with a Chinese soup spoon. What a nutritious first course, and, being liquid, it also slows down the amount of cocktails consumed in the hour! I think she must be a genius.

30-MINUTE POWER RICE AND BEANS

■ SERVES 4.

When we go to visit my fun aunt Elaine, she always has something interesting, delicious, and healthy for us to eat, like this protein-powerful recipe. It's a perfect high-energy meal for families.

1 Mexican chorizo sausage (approx. 8 ounces) (I like to use chicken sausages by Amylu)
2 tablespoons of low-fat olive oil
1 tablespoon of chopped garlic
1 medium onion, chopped
1 red pepper, chopped
1 can (15 ounces) of black or red beans
1 can (about 4 ounces) of corn (optional)
2 cups cooked brown rice

1. Heat a skillet over medium heat. Remove the sausage from casing into the skillet; break it up with a spatula as it cooks. Cook thor-

oughly for 5 to 8 minutes. Drain and set sausage aside, keeping it warm.

2. Wipe out the pan, then sauté the garlic and onions in oil for 5 minutes. Add chopped pepper and cook until tender (about 5 minutes). Add the sausage, beans, and optional corn. Continue cooking until everything is heated through. Stir in the rice and lightly toss until everything is steamy and well blended. Serve immediately.

NOTE: Tonight, prepare the kale for tomorrow's lunch, which needs to marinate overnight.

DAY FOURTEEN

Breakfast

► Grandma Pancakes*

GRANDMA PANCAKES

■ **MAKES ABOUT 10 TO 12 THIN PANCAKES.**

Every Real Mom can be the hero when she makes this special Grandma Pancakes recipe, which is actually a recipe for crepes, handed down to me by my father, Dave—he inherited it from his mother (who was, of course, my grandma Emerson). Add your favorite fruit or nut spread.

Canola oil (for the pan)
1 cup flour
¾ cup milk
1 teaspoon vanilla
3 eggs
Honey (but I like to use agave nectar) to taste

1. Heat an omelet pan or skillet over medium-high heat. Coat lightly with canola oil. In a Vitamix or other blender, combine flour, milk, vanilla, eggs, and honey or agave nectar. Pour a 4-inch circle of batter into the hot pan. Immediately swirl the batter in a circular motion to thinly spread the batter in the pan, making it into about an 8-inch circle. Let the pancake cook until tiny bubbles form on the surface.

2. Using a large spatula, quickly flip the pancake over and cook the other side. The first pancake will be your tester, so don't use too much batter on that one. Set the cooked crepes on a plate covered by a slightly damp paper towel to keep them warm until ready to eat.

Roll fruit, Nutella, or Truwhip in the center for a breakfast surprise "in the middle."

Midmorning Snack

- ▶ For a light and refreshing snack while working in the yard or enjoying the sunshine in the summer, I sun-brew green and hibiscus tea in a glass pitcher and add the juice of a whole lemon. Then I pour it into ice-cube trays to make homemade raw frozen treats.

- ▶ You can also enjoy some fresh fruit with your "tea" treats—1 cup of sliced pineapple, blueberries, and walnuts.

FEED YOUR SPIRIT:
Love Your Mother!

FEEL THE SUN on your face; Mother Nature is amazing. . . . But of course she is. She's a mother.

- ▶ Orange Sesame Kale*
- ▶ 1 cup Double-duty Chicken Soup that you made yesterday, for lunch

ORANGE SESAME KALE

■ SERVES 4.

My sweet and dedicated friend Robyn O'Brien, author of the revealing book *The Unhealthy Truth* and founder of www.allergykidsfoundation.org, shared this recipe! *Yum.*

2 bunches kale
2 cups orange juice
1 cup unsweetened soy milk
1 cup raw tahini (pureed sesame seeds)
½ cup currants
½ teaspoon fresh lemon juice
½ tablespoon unhulled sesame seeds

1. The night before you will eat this, remove large stems from kale and discard. Chop leaves and place in a large bowl. Pour orange juice over the top. Toss to combine. Cover and place in refrigerator overnight.

2. The next day, steam orange juice–soaked kale until tender. In a food processor or powerful blender (like a Vitamix), combine soy milk, tahini, currants, and lemon juice. Blend until smooth and creamy. Toss kale with half of the tahini sauce and sprinkle with sesame seeds.

NOTE: The remaining sauce may be used over steamed Swiss chard, spinach, or any type of greens you desire. Keep it in the fridge and dip raw veggies in it whenever you get the munchies.

Afternoon Snack

- ► Bake up two sweet potatoes (slit the tops and spread some coconut oil on top), slice them up, and eat them as snacks all week, starting today.

- ► 12 salted, roasted cashews (or try raw cashews— they're good)

Dinner

- ► Arugula, Roasted Cherry Tomatoes, & Bocconcini Salad*

ARUGULA, ROASTED CHERRY TOMATOES, & BOCCONCINI SALAD

■ SERVES 4.

When I hosted a Real Moms Love to Eat cooking event with Megan Calhoun's SocialMoms.com, we had the pleasure of cooking with celebrity chef Tyler Florence via UStream. It was way cool! Here's one of the recipes he shared with us.

32 cherry tomatoes, on vine
¼ cup olive oil
2 cloves garlic, thinly sliced
4 sprigs fresh thyme leaves

Sea salt and pepper to taste
6 cups lightly packed baby arugula or baby spinach leaves
¾ cup Wish-Bone Italian dressing
24 bocconcini (fresh mozzarella cheese balls)
½ cup fresh basil leaves
2 cups diced grilled chicken or 4 chicken breasts

NOTE: I added this to the recipe to make it more substantial for dinner, but it's optional—you can buy precooked grilled chicken in the store to save time, or grill it yourself with barbecue sauce, such as Annie's Naturals, which contains no high-fructose corn syrup. Or grill chicken breasts and serve them separately.

1. Preheat oven to 350 degrees. Arrange tomatoes in roasting pan, then drizzle with olive oil. Add garlic and thyme. Season with sea salt and pepper. Roast 15 minutes or until tomatoes are tender and starting to burst.

2. Toss arugula with Wish-Bone Italian dressing in large bowl. Arrange arugula on serving platter, then top with tomatoes and bocconcini. Garnish with basil leaves. Season, if desired, with sea salt and pepper. Optionally, top with diced or whole grilled chicken breast. Enjoy!

BANANA ILLUSION ICE "CREAM"

Freeze a couple of peeled bananas in a freezer bag (wrapped in waxed paper). Blend bananas in a Vitamix blender until fluffy. Scoop and serve as a frozen dessert! You can mix in a couple of strawberries, blueberries, or peach slices to make different flavors.

DAY FIFTEEN

Breakfast

▶ Beth's Best Poached Eggs with Hollandaise Sauce*

▶ 1 piece of Ezekiel toast topped with a light spread of peanut butter

▶ 1 sliced kiwi and 4 strawberries

BETH'S BEST POACHED EGGS WITH HOLLANDAISE SAUCE

■ SERVES 1.

This is a perfect meal for a family Sunday brunch.

2 poached eggs topped with wilted (steamed) spinach and hollandaise sauce
Hollandaise Sauce* (my mom's recipe)
1½ tablespoons of cornstarch
⅔ cup rice milk
1 teaspoon organic butter
Juice of 1 medium lemon
About ⅛ to ¼ teaspoon sea salt
1 egg yolk

Put the cornstarch and rice milk in a small saucepan over medium heat. Continue to whisk mixture while cooking—sauce will begin to thicken to desired consistency. Next, add butter and whisk until it is all melted, then slowly pour in the juice of one lemon and the sea salt and whisk it together to blend. Lower the heat and whisk in the egg yolk until the mixture is creamy.

Throw in the Towel—Again

TAKE A COTTON washcloth and run it under hot water; then wring it out. Rub the hot towel over your arms, legs, face, and neck (not necessarily in that order). Refreshing. I suggest this one more than once this month because it is so amazing!

Midmorning Snack

▶ Sahar's Healthy Hummus*

SAHAR'S HEALTHY HUMMUS

You'll love this recipe from Sahar Aker, a veteran TV news health reporter now making videos and writing about diet, fitness, and the obesity epidemic at www.FatFighterTV.com.

15-ounce can garbanzo beans, drained, liquid reserved
1 tablespoon tahini (sesame paste)
1 lemon—squeezed for juice
2 garlic cloves, minced
1 teaspoon cumin
¼ teaspoon cayenne pepper
¼ teaspoon salt
¼ teaspoon paprika
Optional garnishes: a few kalamata olives and a drizzle of olive oil

In food processor, puree garbanzo beans, tahini, lemon juice, and as much garbanzo bean liquid as needed to form a coarse paste. Add seasonings. Blend thoroughly. Transfer to a bowl and sprinkle with a little paprika. Serve with sliced veggies and crackers or pita bread. Top with any garnishes.

Lunch

- ► Garden-to-table Gazpacho*
- ► Optional: a few slices of turkey, ham, or chicken

GARDEN-TO-TABLE GAZPACHO

■ **SERVES 6 TO 8.**

My dear friend Sharon Meyers, who was one of the editors for my online magazine and is a marketing specialist for chefs and restaurants, brings years of living overseas in the Middle East and Asia to her cooking approach and entertaining style. This easy-to-make garden-to-table soup takes just ten minutes to make, if everyone helps!

4 slices bread and water to soak
6 large tomatoes, cut into cubes
2 cloves garlic, peeled
⅓ cup extra virgin olive oil
½ teaspoon each black pepper, ground cumin, and curry powder
2 teaspoons sea salt
2 tablespoons lemon or lime juice
1½ cups cold tomato juice
¼ cup chopped cilantro
1 avocado, cubed

1. Tear bread into chunks and soak it in enough water to cover until softened. Puree tomatoes in blender or food processor, then put aside in separate bowl.

2. Squeeze the water from the bread; put bread into food processor with garlic, and blend until smooth.

3. Add oil in a stream, then spices, tomato puree, and lemon or lime juice. Add tomato juice in a stream to finish blending. Cover and chill in the refrigerator for at least 1 hour, or overnight.

4. Serve cold, garnishing each serving with a bit of chopped cilantro and a few cubes of avocado on top.

Afternoon Snack

- ► Sautéed Spinach*
- ► Poached or hard-boiled egg

SAUTÉED SPINACH

■ SERVES 2 TO 3.

2 teaspoons olive oil
6 cups spinach
Juice from 1 lemon
15-ounce can chickpeas (garbanzo beans), drained and rinsed

Heat a skillet over medium-high heat. Add the olive oil. Add the spinach all at once and toss. When the spinach starts to wilt, squeeze the fresh lemon juice on top. Mix in chickpeas. Stir until heated through. Serve immediately. (Leftovers are also good cold, as a snack.)

FEED YOUR SOUL:
Little Box of Love

DO YOU HAVE a memorabilia box? What's inside? When was the last time you looked inside? If you don't have one, maybe it's time to create one, to store all your favorite silly little nostalgic secret treasures, the things that have meaning only to you—and maybe one or two others.

Dinner

▶ Baked Chicken with Honey and Apples*

▶ Rice or noodles

🍳 BAKED CHICKEN WITH HONEY AND APPLES

■ **SERVES 6.**

I'm so proud to support the organization created by Rochelle Davis, executive director of the Healthy Schools Campaign, an independent, not-for-profit organization that provides a voice for people who care about our environment, our children, and education. She loves to cook this favorite family recipe for her two kids, Emily and Brian.

Rochelle adapted this recipe from one by Ron and Nancy Goor. It's tailor-made for the Jewish holiday of Rosh Hashanah, of which honey and apples are symbolic foods. They represent the hope that the New Year will be sweet, healthy, and happy.

6 organic or pasture-raised boneless, skinless chicken breast
    halves
1 tablespoon olive oil, divided
½ sweet onion, sliced (like Vidalia)
2 organic Granny Smith apples, cored and sliced
1½ cups organic apple juice
2 tablespoons honey
1 teaspoon salt

1. Preheat the oven to 350 degrees. Put the chicken in a shallow baking pan.

2. Heat half the olive oil in a large, deep skillet over medium heat. Add the onions and cook, stirring occasionally, until tender, about 4 minutes. Add the apples and cook for about a minute. Pour over the chicken.

3. Warm the remaining olive oil in the same pan over medium heat. Stir in the apple juice, honey, and salt. Cook, scraping the bottom of the pan, for 2 minutes. Pour over the apples.

4. Bake until bubbly and the chicken is no longer pink in the center, about 45 minutes. Serve with any sauce remaining in the baking pan.

DAY SIXTEEN

Breakfast

▸ Michele's Bacon and Eggs Creation*

MICHELE'S BACON AND EGGS CREATION

■ **SERVES 4.**

Growing up, my sister and I shared a room. We giggled and shared everything from hairbrushes to lipstick. Every Sunday morning, we'd awake to the intoxicating aroma of Dad's bacon cooking in the pan. To this day, my sister and I share a steadfast love for breakfast food, any time of the day. Here is her version of our childhood memory.

4 toasted Rudi's Organic Bakery multigrain English muffins
8 slices Applegate Farms organic turkey bacon, fried
8 eggs, scrambled with a splash of rice milk (or the milk of your choice)
4 tablespoons strawberry jam

Smear a thin layer of jam on each toasted muffin. Place 2 pieces of bacon over the jam, forming an X on top. Scoop the eggs on top of the bacon, dividing between the muffins. Top it off with the other side of the muffin. Dig in!

Take a Leap of Faith

ARE YOU LIVING your passion? It's never to late to learn something new, take a class, take a trip, or take that leap of faith you've always feared, whether it's applying for a new job, starting a band, or finally writing that novel you've been thinking about writing for years. You don't have to transform your life radically to take the first few steps toward your dream. What are you waiting for?

Midmorning Snack

▶ Karina's Get-to-it Power Snack*

KARINA'S GET-TO-IT POWER SNACK

■ **SERVES 1.**

My awesome friend Karina was the woman responsible for encouraging me to study holistic nutrition with her, so naturally, her get-to-it mommy snack is balanced and delicious. It quenches my sweet and protein cravings all in one (plus fiber!).

1 cup fat-free Greek yogurt
2 tablespoons old-fashioned organic oatmeal (dry)
1 banana (mash it up so it gets stuck to all of the other ingredients)
½ cup berries (can be any type, but I love blueberries)
1 whole piece of chopped fruit (whatever is in season—an apple, nectarine, peach . . .)
10 almonds (raw)
5 walnuts (raw)
Dash of cinnamon
OPTIONAL: 1 tablespoon organic peanut butter

Mix all ingredients with a fork; then use that fork to gobble them up.

Lunch

- ▶ The Go-To Mom's Chicken and Veggies All in One*
- ▶ Steamed rice or whole-grain toast

FEED YOUR BODY:
Sitting Pretty

SITTING UPRIGHT IN a chair, inhale as you pull your shoulders back as if you are trying to bring your shoulder blades together. Hold that stretch for five seconds and release. Repeat.

THE GO-TO MOM'S CHICKEN AND VEGGIES ALL IN ONE

■ SERVES 4.

You get to choose the amounts of veggies, making this a no-pressure meal.

I love Kimberley Baine and her Go-To Mom's Quick & Easy All in One Recipe—or as she sometimes calls it, "the Lazy Mom Meal"! When she's not busy filming segments for Go-To Mom TV or MommytoMommy.TV, she's giving expert professional advice as a national child development expert and licensed child therapist.

5 chicken breasts
Sliced onions (as many as you choose)
Broccoli pieces (as many as you choose)
Baby carrots (as many as you choose)
½ cup (or more) Wish-Bone Italian salad dressing

Preheat the oven to 350 degrees. Rinse chicken and pat dry. Place chicken in a glass baking dish. Add vegetables around and on the chicken. Pour salad dressing over everything. Cover tightly with foil and bake for 30 minutes.

Serve with steamed rice or whole-grain toast; save one breast for tomorrow's lunch!

Afternoon Snack

▶ Baked Winter Squash*

BAKED WINTER SQUASH

■ **SERVES 4 TO 6 SIDES.**

You'll have leftovers after making this—makes a great snack throughout the week!

2 or 3 winter squash, such as acorn or butternut

Cut the squash in half and scoop out the seeds (discard or roast them later). Put about half an inch of water in a baking pan. Place the squash, cut sides down, in the water. Bake for 30 to 45 minutes, or until squash flesh is easily pierced with a fork. Cool and scoop out the flesh. Discard the skins. Enjoy a small bowl of the mashed flesh with a drizzle of olive oil or butter and salt and pepper or, for a sweeter version, with a bit of butter, cinnamon, and nutmeg.

Dinner

▶ Seared Scallops with Cucumber Salad*

SEARED SCALLOPS WITH CUCUMBER SALAD

■ **SERVES 2 TO 4.**

Some nights you may want to eat a lighter dinner; tonight's one of those nights for me.

This lip-smacking recipe comes from my way-cool friend and fellow Integrative Nutrition student Frank Giglio, holistic chef and owner of Frank's Finest. Frank is also the executive chef and contributing editor for thebestdayever. com.

1 large English cucumber
1 cup snap peas, cut into thirds
2 tablespoons thinly sliced red onion
¼ cup fresh dill, roughly chopped
1 to 2 tablespoons olive oil
2 to 3 teaspoons apple cider vinegar
Sea salt to taste
Freshly cracked black peppercorns
8 large scallops
A sprinkle of Frank's Finest lemon-pepper blend (or other favorite seasoning)
2 tablespoons coconut oil
½ lemon for drizzling
1 green onion, top sliced thin

1. With a mandoline or sharp knife, thinly slice the cucumber. Place into a large bowl; mix in the snap peas, onions, and dill. Drizzle in the olive oil and vinegar, then season with sea salt and freshly cracked black pepper. Toss well and allow flavors to meld.

2. Place the scallops on a dish and season with lemon-pepper blend. Heat a large, heavy-bottomed skillet over medium-high heat. Melt the coconut oil and, when a light amount of smoke is visible, add the scallops. Cook on one side until well browned; then flip each scallop, turn off the heat, and allow to rest in the pan for 1 to 2 minutes before removing.

3. Place a small amount of cucumber salad onto 2 plates. Place 4 scallops around each salad. Drizzle the plate with lemon juice and sliced green onions. Serve and enjoy!

BANANA FROZEN DREAM

What could be simpler? Take frozen bananas and whip them up in the Vitamix blender until fluffy, scoop out, and serve as a frozen treat. Sprinkle in a teaspoon of raw cacao powder before blending, for a chocolate-banana-dream version.

DAY SEVENTEEN

Breakfast

- ▶ A+ Plan Summer Fruit Salad*
- ▶ 2 hard-boiled eggs

A+ PLAN SUMMER FRUIT SALAD

When I met Amanda Winters, the founder of A+ Plan Nutrition & Style Consulting, she told me about this tasty fruit salad. I love it so much, I often eat it for breakfast, but you can also make this beautiful, colorful, and superhealthy fruit salad for barbecues, or just to keep around the house for your family to munch on.

Simply combine sliced pink grapefruit, strawberries, watermelon, yellow apples, nectarines, kiwi, and peaches in any amount (or substitute the fruits you have on hand). Add a handful of organic coconut flakes and a drizzle of lemon juice and mix it all together.

The coconut flakes not only add taste and texture but have beneficial properties for cleansing and support of the nervous system and the thyroid gland, among other benefits. The lemon juice not only prevents the apple from turning color, but it also balances out the sweetness with a tart flavor.

Feel free to experiment and add different treats, depending on the occasion. Add some nuts or seeds and yogurt for a great breakfast, or some chocolate chips to make it a dessert. It's your fruit salad, so enjoy it the way *you like it*!

FEED YOUR SOUL :
Your Own Picasso

I LOVE TO paint. I'm no Picasso, but I really enjoy painting. It's fun and relieves my stress. Why not try your hand at it too? Purchase some paints and an easel and see where your spirit takes you.

Midmorning Snack

▶ Kaleberry Smoothie*

KALEBERRY SMOOTHIE

■ SERVES 2.

This recipe is contributed by Bernadette Penotti.

1 cup blueberries (frozen or fresh)
1 large ripe Fuji apple (or any kind of apple), cored
5 large leaves of kale ("spines" removed)
1 cup filtered water or coconut water

Blend in a Vitamix or other blender and drink immediately. Surprisingly tasty!

Lunch

▶ Pancetta Pea Soup*

PANCETTA PEA SOUP

■ **SERVES 8.**

My friend and fellow student at the Institute for Integrative Nutrition Mishra H. Keller is a certified holistic health counselor and the founder and director of Nutrisults, where she specializes in helping women who are tired of dieting experience weight loss and increased energy, and feel good in their bodies again. She's also a new mother.

1 pound dried split peas
1 tablespoon olive oil
5 slices pancetta, chopped (or use lean ham)
7 cloves garlic, minced
½ large onion, chopped
6 cups filtered water
3 bay leaves
4 teaspoons salt

1. Sort and rinse peas. In a large soup pot or Dutch oven, heat the oil. Add pancetta and cook on medium-high heat until crispy. Add garlic and onions and cook for 3 to 4 minutes. Stir in the peas. Add water and bay leaves. Bring to a boil, then cover and simmer for 30 to 45 minutes, or until peas are tender.

2. Add salt, stir, remove bay leaves and then serve.

FEED YOUR BODY:
Nostalgia Fitness

REMEMBER IN GRADE school how they had the physical fitness tests? How many sit-ups can you do (the old-fashioned ones, not the yuppie-on-a-ball kind)? How about pull-ups? Can you do one? Two? Or ten? Let's work on it together.

Afternoon Snack

► Corn on the cob is delicious cold with a light sprinkle of olive oil and sea salt or pepper

► 2 Organic Valley Stringles or 2 pieces of any string cheese

► ½ cup organic red grapes

Dinner

► Meat Loaf and More*

► Noodles or mashed potatoes

► Green Beans Almandine*

MEAT LOAF AND MORE

My friend Renee Iseson, who is a lover of wine and chocolate—and would rather have dessert first—calls herself an executive chef for three little people who each have his or her own taste buds. She's a Work at Home Mom (WAHM) who was a former advertising and marketing executive.

This is not your mother's meat loaf! Remember the chopped meat formed into a ball and baked? Dry and flavorless. Well, this meat loaf is packed full of healthy veggies and is exceptionally moist and flavorful! It's my kids' favorite. It has become a staple in our house and it can be in yours too!

INGREDIENTS, PART 1:

2 tablespoons unsalted butter or margarine or extra virgin olive oil

¾ cup minced onion

½ cup minced celery

½ cup minced carrot

¼ cup minced red bell pepper

2 teaspoons minced garlic
1 large handful fresh spinach, chopped (you can use frozen
      too—1 small package)
Small jalapeño, minced, for added kick (optional)

INGREDIENTS, PART 2:
1 teaspoon salt
¼ teaspoon cayenne pepper
½ teaspoon black pepper
½ teaspoon ground cumin
½ teaspoon nutmeg
½ cup half-and-half
½ cup organic ketchup (look for the kind without high-fructose
      corn syrup)
2 eggs, beaten (or Egg Beaters, equivalent to two eggs)
2 pounds lean ground beef
½ to ¾ cup dry bread crumbs
Additional organic ketchup for topping the meat loaf

1. Preheat the oven to 375 degrees.

2. Melt the butter in a large pan. Add all of the remaining ingredients from part 1. Sauté until vegetables are soft. Set aside to cool.

3. In a large bowl combine the part 2 ingredients. Mix together well, adding the bread crumbs last. Add just enough to get a mixture that binds together and isn't too mushy.

4. Shape the meat into a loaf and place in a loaf pan. Create a shallow indentation down the middle of the loaf and fill with a line of organic ketchup.

5. Bake 1½ to 2 hours. It should be brown on top but not burned.

6. There may be a lot of liquid (extra fat) in the pan after it's cooked, depending on how lean your meat was. Remove the meat loaf from pan to a plate with a slotted spatula, drain the liquid, and put the meat loaf back in the pan for easy cleanup. Serve warm with noodles or mashed potatoes.

GREEN BEANS ALMANDINE

4 ounces sliced almonds
1 tablespoon olive oil
1½ pounds green beans
Sea salt and pepper, to taste

In a skillet over medium heat, lightly sauté almonds in 1 tablespoon of olive oil; watch them to be sure they don't burn. Steam green beans; then toss with the almonds and season with sea salt and pepper before serving.

Optional Dessert

▶ Slinky, Sultry Raw Chocolate Mousse* (See the recipe on page 97)

DAY EIGHTEEN

Breakfast

▶ Wendy's Welsh Cakes*

▶ Green Smoothie

WENDY'S WELSH CAKES

■ **SERVES 6 TO 8.**

Wendy Walker was the editor of the book *Chicken Soup for the Soul: Power Moms,* my publishing debut. After a successful career as a lawyer, she wrote the books *Four Wives* and *The Queen of Suburbia.* Her recipe hits the spot on a chilly morning.

1 cup organic whole-wheat flour

¼ cup organic butter

¼ teaspoon salt

¼ cup organic sugar (can substitute ¹⁄₁₆ teaspoon liquid stevia
   sweetener)

1 tablespoon baking powder

½ teaspoon baking soda

½ to 1 cup buttermilk (enough liquid to make a soft dough)

1 organic egg

¼ to ½ cup organic raisins (depending upon taste)

Blend the butter into the flour and salt. Add the other dry ingredients and mix well. Add the milk and egg to make a soft dough and turn on a floured board. Shape into a round and roll to about ½-inch thick and slice (like mini pancakes). Bake both sides on a hot skillet (or you can bake in the oven at 350 degrees—they come out like scones). Add a small dab of butter and enjoy.

Midmorning Snack

▶ Peanut Butter–Banana Rollups*

▶ Organic Low-fat Blueberry Kefir Smoothie drink
   (found in most grocery stores)

PEANUT BUTTER-BANANA ROLLUPS*

As a busy working mom, the last thing my good friend Teri Knapp will do in the morning is eat breakfast. She makes her two teenagers a protein-loaded breakfast—special-order for each—and packs their lunches so they can avoid the school cafeteria. Once they are out the door, so is she. She shared with me that she'll often take an organic tortilla, spread it with peanut butter, lay a banana down, and wrap it up. It's mess-free to eat on the go and keeps her full for quite a while. There is something about peanut butter that keeps the hunger pangs away. Go, Teri!

FEED YOUR RELATIONSHIPS:
Smile, Say Cheese

SNAP SOME PICTURES today of people and places you love; then print and post them on a bulletin board where you can see them, or upload them to your computer desktop or screen saver.

Lunch

► Greens, reds, yellows and purples. Chop up all of your favorite vegetables (and maybe a few pieces of fruit) and top with some nuts of your choice. Mix it all together with some of the Orange Sesame Dressing on page 216.)

Afternoon Snack

► Sliced heirloom tomatoes and thinly sliced basil seasoned with sea salt and a drizzle of olive oil and balsamic vinegar

► Large glass of green hibiscus tea sweetened with stevia on the side (just a pinch—this sweetener has kick!)

FEED YOUR BODY:
Time to Play Footsie, Again:

GET A GOOD footbath and keep it where you'll see and use it. Fill it up with warm water and maybe drop in a few drops of scented oils. Dip your toes, then your feet in; exhale and sit quietly for five minutes. Have more time? Then take it—just pull your tootsies out when the water starts to get cold.

Dinner

► Warm Chevre Salad*

WARM CHEVRE SALAD

■ SERVES 4.

> I love how Leonard Hollander, executive chef of Marion Street Cheese Market, creates dishes rooted in local and seasonal ingredients that also reflect the café's mission statement, created with a sense of whimsy and the desire to make diners comfortable. He brings culinary arts experience to this Oak Park location via previous work in Cincinnati, Los Angeles, and Chicago.

½ cup orange juice
½ cup water
1 cup golden raisins
1 small head of fennel, very thinly sliced
12 ounces mixed greens (spinach, baby romaine, red oak, red leaf, mizuna, etc.)
4 warm Chevre medallions—recipe follows
½ cup citrus vinaigrette—recipe follows
1 teaspoon kosher salt

1. In a small saucepan over medium heat, bring the orange juice and water to a simmer and add the raisins. Remove from the heat and allow the mixture to cool to room temperature. Strain the liquid off and reserve the raisins.

To serve:

2. In a large bowl, toss together the fennel, raisins, and greens. Season lightly with salt and pour dressing over the mixture; toss to combine. Divide between four plates and place a warm goat cheese medallion on top.

CITRUS VINAIGRETTE
Juice and zest of 1 lemon, 1 lime, 1 orange
1 tablespoon local honey
1 teaspoon whole-grain mustard
1 shallot, minced

2 tablespoons white balsamic vinegar (substitute white wine or
   champagne vinegar)
¾ cup grape-seed oil
Kosher salt to taste

Combine the citrus juices and zest in a medium bowl, add the
honey, mustard, shallot, and vinegar. While whisking slowly,
stream in the grape-seed oil and season to taste.

WARM CHEVRE MEDALLIONS
½ cup flour
1 teaspoon salt
½ cup buttermilk
1 egg
3 ounces finely chopped hazelnuts
6 ounces chevre (fresh goat cheese, like Capriole)

1. To set up a breading station, get 3 small bowls. In one, put the
flour and salt. In the next, put buttermilk and egg, whisked together. In the last, put the hazelnuts.

2. Preheat the oven to 375 degrees. Divide the goat cheese into 4 equal
parts. Shape each piece into a small puck-shaped medallion and roll
in the flour to coat. Dip each one into the buttermilk-and-egg mixture, rubbing lightly to ensure that they are entirely coated. Last, toss
each ball in the hazelnuts and press to reshape. Place on a small baking sheet and bake for 6 to 8 minutes, or until nuts are toasted.

3. Feel free to add a side of sliced roasted chicken breast, to include
a little extra protein.

EARTH LOVE:
Herbalicious!

PLACE LITTLE POTS of fresh growing herbs on your kitchen countertop, in front of a window. Water daily and you'll have fresh herbs
at your fingertips whenever you need them. I like to keep rosemary,
basil, and chives growing in my kitchen. What herbs do you like?

DAY NINETEEN

Breakfast

- ► Bird in a Nest*
- ► ½ cup blueberries and raspberries
- ► Green hibiscus tea seasoned with stevia

🍳 BIRD IN A NEST

■ **SERVES 1.**

I love making this fancy little breakfast. Just make as many as you need. For each serving, using a biscuit or cookie cutter, cut out a 2-inch circle from the center of a piece of good bread (I like French Meadow Man's Bread). Lightly spray a frying pan with organic cooking spray. Fry one egg inside the biscuit cutter. Steam or sauté several leaves of spinach; then place them atop the circle of bread. Place the cooked fried egg on top of the cooked spinach. Season with sea salt and pepper. Enjoy your Bird in a Nest!

Midmorning Snack

- ► Kashi caramel-peanut GOLEAN® Roll (This snack bar has a chewy nougat center rolled in whole grains, nuts, and crisps)
- ► Sliced fruit

FEED YOUR BODY:
Breathe

JUST BREATHE . . . in through the nose . . . out through the mouth . . . as you slowly say, "Hhhaaa." Repeat several times—easy does it.

- ▶ Roasted Red Beet Soup*
- ▶ 2 slices of Applegate Farms roast beef, rolled up

ROASTED RED BEET SOUP

■ **SERVES 4.**

This colorful and tasty recipe is from the founders of MapleSyrupWorld.com. The site provides a selection of hand-selected, high-quality maple products and a community portal of free information and recipes relating to maple syrup. More than just pancakes!

1 bunch of small beets
Extra virgin olive oil
1 medium-size onion, chopped
2 small garlic cloves, minced
½-inch piece of ginger, minced
Zest of 1 orange
Pinch of chili powder
1 cup vegetable broth
Juice of 3 oranges (or about 1 cup)
1 tablespoon maple syrup
Sea salt and pepper, to taste

OPTIONAL: 3 tablespoons crème fraîche

1. Preheat the oven to 375 degrees.

2. Cut the greens off the beets, scrub the beets clean, and place them on a large sheet of aluminum foil. Drizzle with olive oil and fold the foil over, creating a closed pouch. Roast until tender. Depending on the number and size, this should take 30 to 45 minutes. Remove the beets from the oven and let them cool enough for you to peel them with your fingers. Cut them into large cubes.

3. In a large skillet, heat 2 tablespoons of olive oil over medium heat and sauté the onion for about 3 minutes. Add the garlic, ginger, orange zest, and a pinch of chili powder and sauté for another minute.

4. Add beet cubes and broth, bring the liquid to a boil, and let it simmer for 10 to 15 minutes, or until the beets are extremely soft.

5. Use a hand mixer or transfer the vegetables to a food processor, add orange juice, and purée to a smooth, velvety consistency.

6. Add maple syrup and season with sea salt and black pepper or some more chili powder, until you find it sweet, salty, or spicy enough.

7. Serve at room temperature or chilled.

OPTIONAL: Add one tablespoon of crème fraîche to each bowl right before serving.

FEED YOUR BODY-MIND-SPIRIT:
Chocolate

NEED A SUPERQUICK chocolate fix? Mix a teaspoon of cocoa powder with a tablespoon of agave nectar. Lick that spoon!

Afternoon Snack

- ► TerrAmazon cacao–macadamia nut snack, 2-ounce pouch
- ► ½ cup berries of your choice

Dinner

- ► Rolled Chicken Breast*
- ► Huge Salad*

ROLLED CHICKEN BREAST

■ **SERVES 4.**

> I can thank my nutritionist, Sherry Belcher, for many
> things: my ongoing health, feeding my constant curiosity
> for food and nutrition, and her support for everything I aim
> to accomplish. Her perpetual belief in me has made me the
> woman I am today. This recipe is from her too.

4 boneless, skinless chicken breast halves
1 cup baby spinach or baby arugula
4 tablespoons chopped sun-dried tomatoes that have been re-
      constituted in water for 5 minutes
4 tablespoons feta or goat cheese
Seasoned salt or salt and pepper
2 tablespoons olive oil
¼ cup chicken stock

1. Pound each chicken breast flat by putting between two sheets of
plastic wrap and using a meat pounder or bottom of a heavy pan.
Sprinkle with sea salt and pepper.

2. Starting at one end of the chicken breast, add ¼ cup spinach
leaves, and 1 tablespoon each tomatoes and cheese. Gently but
tightly roll the chicken breast around the filling and secure with a
toothpick. Sprinkle with seasoned salt or salt and pepper.

3. Heat olive oil over medium heat. Add chicken breasts. Brown on
all sides. Reduce heat to medium-low and add chicken broth. Cover
and cook 20 minutes.

HUGE SALAD

Nothing screams *salad* more than a delicious chicken dish, so grab
a bunch of mixed greens (the greener the better, a large handful for

each person served); then add raw veggies to your heart's content, such as julienned carrots, red onion, sliced roma tomatoes, and sliced green peppers. Sprinkle with sunflower seeds. Toss it all together and top with raspberry vinaigrette dressing (just one tablespoon per serving).

DAY TWENTY

Breakfast

- ► Hubby Scramble*
- ► Pineapples, strawberries, and grapes
- ► Ezekiel whole-wheat or raisin toast

HUBBY SCRAMBLE

■ SERVES AS MANY AS YOU LIKE!

My husband and kids are huge fans of my scrambled eggs. Even with this simple recipe, they keep coming back for more. Hubby loves them with diced turkey bacon and ham. Make as much as you want, using two eggs per person (or more when people are superhungry).

Eggs (2 per person)
Splash of rice milk
1 tablespoon butter
1 ounce each per person of Applegate Farms organic Sunday
    bacon and diced Applegate Farms organic uncured ham (or
    any other bacon and lean ham)

Whisk desired number of eggs with a splash of rice milk (or any milk you prefer). Heat a skillet over medium-high heat. Melt one tablespoon of butter in the skillet and tilt the pan to coat the bottom.

Add about 1 ounce per person served of cooked and chopped Applegate Farms organic Sunday bacon and diced pieces of Applegate Farms organic uncured ham. Stir continuously with a wooden spoon or heat-resistant spatula until the bacon is cooked.

Add the eggs and stir constantly, breaking up the eggs so they don't turn into an omelet. Leave eggs a bit "wet" and turn off the heat. While eggs are sitting in pan, set up your plates with slices of pineapple, strawberries and grapes. Scoop generous spoonfuls of eggs onto each plate. Serve with toast.

FEED YOUR BODY AND SOUL:
Heads Up

GENTLY MASSAGE YOUR hair and scalp. Close your eyes and imagine your troubles melting away with each stroke of your hands.

Midmorning Snack

▶ LÄRABAR, in your favorite flavor

▶ Watermelon juice (in summer)

In the summer, I blend an entire watermelon (cut in chunks, off the rind, to save my blender blade) until it's blended to pure juice (compliments of the überpowerful Vitamix) and store in a glass pitcher for a cleansing and refreshing glass of "summer" juice anytime of the day.

Lunch

▶ Vegetable Shepherd's Pie*

VEGETABLE SHEPHERD'S PIE

■ **SERVES 6.**

I try to plan ahead and make this the night before and have it in the refrigerator to heat up for lunch the next day. Robyn O'Brien, founder of www.allergykidsfoundation.org, shared this recipe with me for the perfect hearty lunch.

4 large sweet potatoes
1 cup chopped broccoli
1 cup chopped cauliflower
1 medium leek, chopped
1 red bell pepper, cut into 1-inch squares
1 teaspoon herbes de Provence (dried French herbs)
4 tablespoons Dr. Fuhrman's VegiZest or other no-salt veggie
    soup base
2 cups water
2 cups chopped organic spinach
½ cup carrot juice
4 teaspoons cornstarch
1 cup firm tofu, water squeezed out, and crumbled
1 cup hazelnuts, Brazil nuts, or almonds, chopped medium-fine
    (optional)
2 tablespoons chopped fresh parsley, for garnish (optional)

Preheat oven to 375 degrees.

1. Bake sweet potatoes until soft, about 45 minutes. When potatoes are tender, remove to a bowl and mash.

2. Add broccoli, cauliflower, leeks, bell peppers, herbes de Provence, and Dr. Fuhrman's VegiZest to a large sauté pan along with 2 cups of water. Simmer until almost tender (about 10 minutes). Stir in spinach and cook until wilted. Drain vegetables, reserving vegetable liquid in pot.

3. Whisk cornstarch into carrot juice and continue to whisk into boiling vegetable liquid until it thickens. Add vegetables and crumbled tofu to sauce and toss to combine.

4. Divide mixture into two 8-inch pie pans. If desired, top with ½ cup nuts. Spread sweet potatoes over the top and sprinkle with remaining nuts if desired.

5. Bake at 375 degrees for 20 to 30 minutes until hot and lightly browned. If desired, sprinkle with parsley.

Frozen chopped broccoli, cauliflower, and spinach may be substituted for fresh. Thaw and drain well. Do not precook.

This dish may be prepared ahead and frozen, unbaked. Cover tightly with aluminum foil before freezing. Do not defrost, but bake an additional 10 to 15 minutes.

Afternoon Snack

► Fruit with built-in handles (bananas, apples, bunch of grapes)

► ¼ cup salted, roasted sunflower seeds (or choose raw seeds, if you like)

FEED YOUR SOUL:
The Power of Water

SIT BY ANY natural body of water, whether ocean, lake, pond, or streambed; let the rhythmic sounds clear your head. In a pinch, a nice fountain in the park or even a goldfish pond will do.

Dinner

► Savvy, Sassy Flank Steak*

► Brown Rice with Bling*

► Small green side salad

SAVVY, SASSY FLANK STEAK

■ **SERVES 4 TO 6.**

I love working with my good friend Liz on Stella & Dot jewelry parties! It's fun to be a hip and savvy Real Mom, and when it comes to making one mean flank steak, she takes the cake!

1½- to 2-pound flank steak

MARINADE:
¼ cup soy sauce (low-sodium)
¼ cup Worcestershire sauce
1 clove garlic, mashed (or 1 teaspoon garlic powder)
1 teaspoon cilantro
1 teaspoon sliced ginger
1 to 2 limes, sliced and juiced
2 green onions, sliced thin

Prick meat so marinade will permeate it. Combine remaining ingredients and place with meat in a covered glass Pyrex dish; marinate in the refrigerator for a few hours or overnight. Remove the meat from the marinade and discard the marinade. Grill to your desired temperature.

BROWN RICE WITH BLING

Josie Maurer is a hungry woman, wife, and mother of four children. She blogs about food and fitness at YumYucky.com. If you think brown rice is healthy but lacks flavor, you'll love her take on this simple rice recipe. Just make enough to serve the people at your table, using the package directions.

Uncooked brown rice
Medium onion

Canned chicken broth
1 teaspoon olive oil

1. Following package directions, measure out desired amount of brown rice.

2. Instead of water, use an equal amount of canned chicken broth. Add broth to rice. Cut onion in 4 quarters and peel. Add onion quarters and olive oil to the pot. Set rice on high until boiling; then simmer on low with the lid slightly open. Be sure to check frequently to prevent overcooking.

3. Remove cooked onions from pot or enjoy in your rice for extra flavor.

Serve with a small side salad—the greener the better—topped with colorful veggies, served with one tablespoon of your choice of dressing.

Optional Dessert

▶ Easy Beanies*

EASY BEANIES

Annie Tierney, a talented and charismatic former intern at my magazine and Web site, loves this recipe and thinks you will too!

1 box organic chocolate brownie mix
1 can organic black beans

Put the black beans in the Vitamix blender and blend until they are liquefied. Stir the beans into a bowl with the dry organic brownie mix. Place mixture in a pan and bake for about 15 minutes; then check for consistency. A toothpick inserted in the center should come out mostly clean, or with moist crumbs but not batter. Enjoy great-tasting brownies with extra fiber!

DAY TWENTY-ONE

Breakfast

► Apple Cobbler du Barbi*

APPLE COBBLER DU BARBI

■ SERVES 2.

My cyberpal Barbi Walker is an award-winning journalist and avid athlete who loves to eat, cook, and travel with her husband and young son. She's my kind of Real Mom.

This is perfect for breakfast or dessert, just for you, or to share with the kids.

¾ cup old-fashioned Quaker oats (you can also use instant, but
    not the flavored kind with the added sugar)
Pinch of sea salt
¼ scoop vanilla whey protein powder
½ cup chopped apple, like Granny Smith or Fuji
1 tablespoon slivered almonds or crushed walnuts
½ teaspoon cinnamon

Cook oatmeal and pinch of sea salt according to package. After oatmeal is cooked, mix in chopped apples and protein powder. Sprinkle with nuts and cinnamon to taste.

NOTE: If you like a sweeter taste, swirl in a spoonful of honey or a drop or two of liquid stevia sweetener.

Midmorning Snack

► Sweet Cinnamon Flax Crackers* (See recipe on page 95).

WRITE DOWN TEN to fifteen words that describe who you are now and how you feel today. Then use ten to fifteen more words to describe yourself or how you might act or feel thirty pounds heavier. Last, use ten to fifteen descriptive adjectives to describe the "you" in the best shape of your life.

Lunch

▶ Gingery Sweet Potatoes and Snap Peas*

▶ Sliced chicken breast

GINGERY SWEET POTATOES AND SNAP PEAS

■ **SERVES 4 TO 6.**

Thanks to our RealMomsLovetoEat.com Web site editor and gingery-sweet gal Daisy Simmons for this superrecipe.

2 sweet potatoes, thinly sliced
2 cloves garlic, crushed
½ tablespoon olive oil
12 ounces sugar snap peas
1 tablespoon minced fresh ginger
½ tablespoon sesame oil

Sauté the sweet potatoes, garlic, and salt and pepper in olive oil over medium heat for about 10 minutes. Add snap peas and ginger, and cook for an additional 5 minutes, or until sweet potatoes are softened to taste. Sprinkle with sesame oil and serve. I sometimes add a sliced chicken breast on the side to give this recipe a little extra protein.

Afternoon Snack

► Make a trail mix yourself and store in mini containers. I like to mix walnuts, cashews, and raisins or dried cranberries with cacao nibs and a pinch of sea salt, but you could use any other nuts, seeds, or dried fruit you like. You could even include cracker bits, pretzels, sesame sticks, or any other healthy nibbling foods. Good purse food.

Dinner

► Erica's Delish Fish*

► Butternut Squash Soup with Crispy Shallot Garnish*

ERICA'S DELISH FISH

■ **SERVES 1 FILLET PER PERSON.**

Erica Diamond, founder of WomenontheFence.com, loves making salmon for her family. It's fast, healthy, and delicious.

3- to 5-ounce salmon fillets

MARINADE:

Olive oil
Splash of balsamic vinegar
Oregano (fresh or dried)
Basil
Squeeze of lemon
Fresh garlic, sliced

In the morning, combine all ingredients, add salmon, and refrigerate. In the evening, broil, barbecue, or bake, and voilà! One delish main course dish! You can use this marinade on halibut too.

BUTTERNUT SQUASH SOUP WITH CRISPY SHALLOT GARNISH

■ **SERVES 8 TO 12.**

Jorj Morgan is a cookbook author, brand advocate, and lifestyle expert whose advice has appeared in regional and national outlets that include the *Wall Street Journal*, the *Washington Post*, and *Reader's Digest*. She's one of my favorite guests from my radio show, "A Balanced Life." We share a love for delicious, nutrient-dense food and a passion for living well. This recipe is one of my favorite soups!

FOR SOUP:

1 tablespoon olive oil
1 large yellow onion, peeled and finely diced, about 1½ cups
2 medium carrots, peeled, trimmed, and chopped, about 1 cup
3 medium celery ribs, sliced, about 1 cup
4 medium garlic cloves, peeled and minced, about 1 tablespoon
Salt and freshly ground pepper
1 large butternut squash, peeled and diced, about 6 cups (see note below)
1 large russet potato, peeled and diced, about 1½ cups
2 cups dry white wine
2 quarts homemade chicken broth, or low-sodium chicken broth

2 to 3 sprigs sage leaves
1 large orange, cut in half

NOTE: The best way to cut and peel a butternut squash is to trim off the bottom first, so you have a flat surface and the squash doesn't roll around under your sharp knife! Cut the squash in half, and then in half again. Smaller pieces are easier to handle. Use a vegetable peeler to remove the outer skin. Use a tablespoon to scoop out the seeds (you can save these and roast them later, if you like—good to add to that trail mix you just made!). Now wash the knife and your hands well. The squash is slippery. A clean knife and hands will make chopping easier. Cut it into 1- to 2-inch pieces.

FOR SHALLOTS:
4 large shallots, peeled and thinly sliced, about 1 cup
2 cups canola oil

Heat the olive oil in a large soup pot over medium-high heat. Add the onion, carrots, celery, and garlic to the pot. Cook until the vegetables are soft, about 10 minutes. Season with salt and pepper.

Add the butternut squash and potato to the pot and stir. Pour in the wine and simmer for about 5 minutes. Pour in the stock. Place the sage into the pot. Squeeze the juice of the orange into the pot and add the orange halves. Cook until the vegetables are very soft, about 35 to 40 minutes.

Cool the soup. Remove the sage sprigs and orange halves. Use an immersion blender, food processor, or blender to emulsify the soup. Pour the soup back into the pot and season with salt and pepper.

Place the shallots and the oil in a small pot. Bring to a boil over medium-high heat. Reduce the heat to low and simmer. Turn the onions every few minutes until golden brown, about 15 to 20 minutes. Remove the shallots with a slotted spoon to a dish layered with paper towels. As the shallots sit, they will become crispy. Season with salt and pepper. If not using immediately keep warm in a warming drawer, or in the oven on the lowest setting.

Ladle the soup into bowls or mugs. Top with crispy shallots.

NOTE: This soup is fairly mild, so if you like a spicier squash soup, feel free to spice it up with savory-and-sweet favorites like cumin, chili powder, curry, cinnamon, and ginger.

IS IT REALLY THE END?

Alas . . . could it be our time together is at an end? But no! Perish the thought. Because Real Moms always stick together, and even when they are far apart, they always share a bond.

I hope you've enjoyed our time together as much as I have, and I hope even more fervently that you will continue to enjoy more of the beautiful food the planet has to offer, and that you will teach your children to find both health and pleasure from their food, too. Take what you like from this book, and share what you will—follow the concepts that are laid out for you, and I promise you will feel a beautiful change in your life.

Those who have contributed these recipes have done so with love in their hearts and a genuine interest in supporting your healthy love affair with food, but I know there are many more Real Moms out there with recipes and ideas near and dear to their own hearts. I'd love to hear from you and find out what you thought of these recipes and this book. What would you like to see next? And if you have wonderful, vibrant, life-enhancing recipes of your own that you'd like to share, please send them along. You never know—they could end up in our next book!

In the meantime, eat well, love your family, and most of all, love yourself, in every way—body, mind, and spirit.

Bon Appétit, Real Moms!

Love,
Beth

RealMomsLovetoEat.com

(Please sign up for my free newsletter and blog feeds and send me your recipe!)

Resource Guide

FOOD PRODUCTS

Amy's organic tomato basil pasta sauce: www.amys.com

Annie's Naturals barbecue sauce: www.anniesnaturals.com

Applegate Farms: www.applegatefarms.com

Babybel Cheese: www.mini-babybel.com

Barilla: http://www.barillaus.com/Pages/Home.aspx

Bell & Evans's prepackaged frozen chicken breasts: http://www.
bellandevans.com/frozen

Bragg Liquid Aminos: http://www.bragg.com/

Capriole chevre: http://www.capriolegoatcheese.com/

Chicken sausages by Amylu: http://atkfoods.com/brands/
sausagesbyamylu/

Chocolate whey protein powder: http://www.designerwhey.com/
designer-whey/store-finder.htm

Clif Bars: www.clifbar.com

David Wolfe's raw cacao powder: www.sunfood.com

Dr. Fuhrman's VegiZest: http://www.drfuhrman.com/shop/vegizest.
aspx

Dreamfields pasta: www.dreamfieldsfoods.com/index.php

Earthbound Farm prepackaged organic mini carrots and ranch
dip: www.ebfarm.com

Ezekiel organic sprouted whole-grain flourless bread: http://www.
    foodforlife.com/
French Meadow Bakery: http://www.frenchmeadow.com/
Green & Black's: www.greenandblacks.com/us
Herbamare: http://www.avogel.ca/en/shop/health_food/
    herbamare_orig.php
Ian's Natural Foods whole-wheat panko crumbs: http://www.
    iansnaturalfoods.com/
Kashi Organic Promise Autumn Wheat: www.kashi.com
LÄRABAR: http://www.larabar.com/
Lifeway Kefir Discover: www.lifeway.net
Lucuma powder: www.sunfood.com
Luna & Larry's Coconut Bliss: http://coconutbliss.com
LUNA protein bars: www.lunabar.com/
Maple syrup: www.MapleSyrupWorld.com
Mary's Gone Crackers all-grain, gluten-free crackers: www.
    marysgonecrackers.com
Mrs. Dash seasoning: http://www.mrsdash.com/
Natural nut butter: www.justinsnutbutter.com
Nutella: http://www.nutellausa.com/
Quaker old-fashioned oats: http://www.quakeroats.com/products/
    oatmeal/old-fashioned-oats.aspx
Organic agave nectar: http://www.madhavahoney.com/
    AgaveNectar.aspx
Organic Valley Family of Farms: http://www.organicvalley.coop
Pacific Natural Foods: http://www.pacificfoods.com/
Roland Feng Shui maki rolls seaweed-wrapped rice crackers:
    http://www.rolandfoods.com/#Ul44u8rMD
Rudi's honey-wheat bread: www.rudisbakery.com
Rustic Crust Old World ready-to-bake pizza crust: http://www.
    rusticcrust.com/ready-made-pizza-crust.html
Spectrum extra virgin olive oil cooking spray: http://www.
    spectrumorganics.com/?id=89
Spice House smoked paprika: http://www.thespicehouse.com/
    spices/spanish-smoked-sweet-paprika-pimenton-de-la-vera-
    dulce
Stevia sweetener: http://www.stevia.com/
Stonyfield Farm organic fat-free yogurt: www.stonyfield.com
Tera's Whey's rBGH-free vanilla whey: www.teraswhey.com

TerrAmazon cacao: www.terramazon.com

ThinkThin Bites mini bar: www.thinkproducts.com

Truwhip: http://www.truwhip.com/

Udo's 3-6-9 Oil: http://www.udoerasmus.com/products/oil_blend_
en.htm

Vosges gourmet chocolate: www.vosgeschocolate.com

Whole Foods Market 365 Organic turkey jerky: http://www.
wholefoodsmarket.com/

Wish-Bone salad dressing: http://www.wish-bone.com/tyler/videos/
easy-flavorful-salad.aspx

ZonePerfect nutrition bars and pastas: www.ZonePerfect.com

HELPFUL PEOPLE

Sahar Aker, veteran TV news health reporter, now making videos
and writing about diet, fitness, and the obesity epidemic: www.
FatFighterTV.com

Amanda Winters, founder of the A+ Plan Nutrition & Style
Consulting: www.aplusplan.com

Carolyn Ash, friend, author and skin expert: www.carolynash.com

Denise Austin, celebrity fitness guru: http://www.deniseaustin.com/
publicsite/funnel/index.aspx

Tanya Bennett, mother of two, writer, and musician: www.
ishouldbenapping.com, www.mamabrain.com

Kimberley Baine, GoToMom TV or MommytoMommy.TV,
national child development expert and licensed child therapist:
www.TheGoToMom.com

Sherry Belcher, my nutritionist and author of *Simply Good:
Healthy and Easy Recipes*: www.sherrybelcher.com

Bonita Kindle, friend, raw chef, fitness expert: www.
RawFoodsAndFitness.com

Megan Calhoun: SocialMoms.com

Noel Chapman, Noel's Kitchen Tips blog: www.noelskitchentips.com

Sarah Copeland, writer, urban gardener, passionate cook, and
curator of good living: www.edibleliving.com

Rochelle Davis, founding executive director of Healthy Schools
Campaign: www.HealthySchoolsCampaign.org

Jessica Denay, founder of Hot Moms Club and author of the Hot
Mom Handbook series of books: www.HotMomsClub.com

Erica Diamond, founder of Women on the Fence: www.
WomenOnTheFence.com

Heather Dominic, friend and founder of the EnergyRICH
Entrepreneur Success: www.energyrichcoach.com

Gaylon Emerzian, Emmy Award–winning documentary filmmaker
and cookbook writer: www.Spatulatta.com

Deborah Enos, "One-Minute Wellness Coach": www.
DeborahEnos.com

Brittany Ferrin and Vaidotas Karsokas, executive chefs of the
Truffleberry Market: www.TruffleberryMarket.com

Tyler Florence, celebrity chef: www.tylerflorence.com

Frank Giglio, friend and fellow Integrative Nutrition student,
holistic chef and owner of Frank's Finest. Frank is also the
executive chef and contributing editor for the Best Day Ever:
http://www.thebestdayever.com/; www.frankgiglio.com

Leonard Hollander, executive chef of Marion Street Cheese
Market: www.marionstreetcheesemarket.com

Renee Iseson: www.KitchenConundrum.com

Karina Heinrich friend and fellow health counselor: www.
dearlandon.wordpress.com

Joël Kazouini, chef, famed for his namesake, Chez Joël Bistro
Francais in Chicago and Casa Nostra Restaurant in Marrakech:
www.chezjoelbistro.com

Mishra H. Keller, friend and fellow student at the Institute for
Integrative Nutrition, certified holistic health counselor, and
founder and director of Nutrisults: www.nutrisults.com

Amy Tara Koch, author of *Bump it Up: Transform Your Pregnancy
Into the Ultimate Style Statement*: http://www.bumpitupstyle.
com/about.html

John La Puma, MD, physician and professionally trained chef in
Santa Barbara, California, guest on my radio show, author of
Chef MD's Big Book of Culinary Medicine; Lifetime television
series host: http://drjohnlapuma.com and http://ChefMD.com

Ivy Larson, author of the *Whole Foods Diet Cookbook*: www.
CleanCuisine.com

Josie Maurer, friend, wife, and mother of four children, blogger:
www.YumYucky.com

Sharon Meyers, communications specialist: www.MeyersScarola.com

Jorj Morgan, cookbook author, brand advocate, and lifestyle expert: www.jorj.com

Robyn O'Brien, author of *The Unhealthy Truth*, and founder of Allergy Kids Foundation: www.allergykidsfoundation.org

Liz Opie, friend, Stella & Dot: www.stelladot.com/sites/liz

Georgia Orcutt, program manager at Oldways: www.oldwayspt.org

Bernadette Penotti, health and fitness consultant and intuitive self-care strategist: https://www.bernadettepenotti.com

Dr. Barry Sears, international expert and author, *The Zone* and eleven other books: www.zonediet.com

Daisy Simmons, writer, friend, Web site editor, and right-hand gal: www.daisysimmons.com

Susie Sondag, friend, raw food and healthy living expert : www.hipgoddess.com

Barbi Walker, cyberpal, award-winning journalist, and avid athlete who loves to eat, cook, and travel with her husband and young son: http://bjwpost.wordpress.com

Wendy Walker, friend, author, and editor of *Chicken Soup for the Soul: Power Moms*: http://wendywalkerbooks.com

Jenniffer Weigel, columnist with the *Chicago Tribune* and author of two books: *Stay Tuned* and *I'm Spiritual, Dammit!*: www.staytunedwithjen.com

PLACES

Frontera, Rick Bayless's restaurant: www.fronterakitchens.com

Karyn's Raw Café: www.karynraw.com

Sprouts Farmers Markets: http://sprouts.com/home.php

Trader Joe's: http://www.traderjoes.com/

Truffleberry Market: http://www.truffleberrymarket.com/

Whole Foods Market: http://www.wholefoodsmarket.com/

WEB SITES AND BOOKS

Eat Well Guide, the guide to find local, sustainable . . . anything: http://www.eatwellguide.org/localguide/

Juicing for Life: A Guide to the Health Benefits of Fresh Fruit and Vegetable Juicing, by Cherie Calbom and Maureen Keane

Silver Palate Cookbook, by Julee Rosso and Sheila Lukins
Sudoku puzzle: http://www.websudoku.com

COOKING PRODUCTS

Food dehydrators: www.fooddehydrators.com
Jack La Lanne's Power Juicer: http://www.powerjuicer.com
Saladacco Spiral Slicer: rawgourmet.com/saladacco-spiral-slicer
Vitamix: http://www.vitamix.com/index.asp
Williams-Sonoma (many kitchen products, such as mandolines and
    Silpat baking liners): www.williams-sonoma.com